The Black Death: a Biological Reappraisal

THE BLACK DEATH

a Biological Reappraisal

GRAHAM TWIGG

SCHOCKEN BOOKS · NEW YORK

First American edition published by Schocken Books 1985
10 9 8 7 6 5 4 3 2 1   85 86 87 88
Copyright © Graham Twigg 1984
All rights reserved
Published by agreement with B. T. Batsford Ltd, London

Library of Congress Cataloging in Publication Data
Twigg, Graham.
    The biology of the Black Death.
    Bibliography: p.
    Includes index.
    1. Black death—Etiology.   2. Black death—Europe—
History.   3. Plague.   I. Title.
RC171.T9   1985   614.4′24   84–14149

Manufactured in Great Britain
ISBN 0–8052–3955–3

Contents

Acknowledgements

I am indebted to many people for giving me their time to discuss various aspects of this book during its preparation. I am especially grateful to my son, John, who has given me much advice on historical matters and who critically reviewed the text and encouraged me throughout the work; to my wife, Mary, for her continued support and for assistance with checking and proof reading; to Phil Jones and Professor Colin Kaplan for advice on bacterial diseases and to my students at Royal Holloway College who discussed my ideas and asked many searching questions. To Joyce Pearson I am indebted for advice on the medieval period and to Mr F. A. Wilford and Stephen Usher for assistance with Latin translations. The illustrations have been drawn by Mrs Sarah Wroot and I am especially grateful to her for the time and care she has given to the task.

Dr David E. Davis of California, who has similar ideas on the Black rat in medieval Europe, has corresponded with me for years on this subject and at his suggestion a small group gathered in October 1981 at the British Museum of Natural History to discuss rats in the Middle Ages. Those present were David Davis, Philip Armitage, James Rackham, John Goodall, Terry O'Connor, Juliet Clutton-Brock, Barbara West and myself. This proved to be a particularly stimulating event and I am grateful to all for their views on the subject. I am especially indebted to Terry O'Connor for access to his unpublished material.

Much of the work has been carried out in Cambridge and I am most grateful to my friend John Clevedon-Brown for his hospitality when working there. I also wish to thank the librarians of the University Library and the Science Periodicals Library, Cambridge for permission to use their facilities. Finally, my sincere thanks are due to Miss Josephine Healey for her admirable typing of the book.

List of figures

List of Tables

Preface

The Black Death continues to attract the attention of scholars and laymen alike: in the last decade and a half there has been a resurgence of interest in this important medieval event. The disease is thought to have been bubonic plague and few would currently dissent from that view. It may therefore be regarded as heresy to suggest that there could be reason for doubting this long held belief, but a careful consideration of the events of the medieval disease outbreak has led me to do so.

As a zoologist carrying out research into those animal diseases which are transmitted to man, termed zoonoses, my interest in plague became focused on the Black Death because of certain features of that epidemic which would be considered atypical of plague as we have known it during this century. My approach has been to take our knowledge of modern plague – particularly the requirements of the rodent and flea carriers – and to compare this basic data with the features of the Black Death, in an attempt to test whether the differences between the two can be explained on the grounds of the variability that we might expect in two outbreaks separated by so long a period, or whether the variation is so great that one must conclude they are two different diseases. I can find little evidence for widespread true plague, and must therefore incline to the latter opinion.

The greater part of this book is concerned with the foregoing analysis. However, it would be shirking the issue to leave the matter there; if the epidemic was not plague then some other disease must be sought as the agent of the Black Death. I have suggested an alternative, one whose biology fits the observed pattern of events, and of contemporary versions too, although the records of the past might reasonably lead us to suspect the presence of several concurrent diseases. These same accounts, it should be noted, have often been used as evidence of bubonic plague.

It is my belief that the existing version of the Black Death has been held too rigidly for too long. I hope that this book will stimulate discussion and research not only into its causation but also into that of subsequent epidemics called 'plague' in the British Isles.

CHAPTER ONE

Plague today and the infective cycle

When a disease affecting man spreads and infects not only the inhabitants of one region or country but those of other countries over a wide geographical area, finally spreading across the continents, it is termed a pandemic, as distinct from an epidemic which affects people on a more local basis. The influenza which went round the world in the years immediately following World War I is a well-known example of a pandemic. The factors which determine the rate of spread of a disease are several, and whereas influenza's method of spreading by airborne droplets ensures the most rapid passage, other diseases, dependent upon intermediate carriers, will progress more slowly. Our knowledge of the causative organisms of bacterial diseases only began in the late nineteenth century with the classical researches of Pasteur, Koch and others, and our understanding of viruses came later still. Where these organisms are carried by wild animal vectors the scholar seeking to understand the causation of past diseases must in addition have an understanding of the biology of vertebrate and invertebrate carrier species.

One disease which has received a great deal of attention is bubonic plague and because this is believed to have been the agent of the fourteenth-century Black Death it is not surprising that most published accounts of that episode have been by historians. The latter have, however, been mainly interested in the social and economic effects of plague outbreaks and less in their causation. Biologists, including medical workers, have confined their attentions primarily to the disease in wild animal vectors, a field of research which is inevitably confined to extant populations and which began over 70 years ago as the importance of plague vectors emerged from the work in India (Plague Research Commission, 1906–17).[1] It was fortunate that the newly emerging information about bacteria came just before bubonic plague spread to many parts of the world and when it was causing heavy loss of life in India in the early part of the twentieth century. The research workers were able to harness the new techniques and knowledge to isolate the bacteria from both human patients and the animal vectors and provide much of the basic information on the biology of bubonic plague.

The Black Death is regarded as a major feature of the history of medieval Europe because of the effects it had on many aspects of life and although it may not have been wholly instrumental in initiating certain changes it was probably important in accelerating some which had already begun. Any disease which is said to have killed one third or more of the population in two or three years must rate as a very important historical event and attract a great deal of comment.

Accounts of the Black Death are numerous and although they range from the lurid, over-dramatised to the scholarly all accept, almost without question, that bubonic plague was the disease responsible for the great fourteenth-century pandemic. There are, indeed, certain features of the symptoms of the Black Death which occur in bubonic plague but they are also evident in some other diseases. Nevertheless, once bubonic plague had been suggested as the factor responsible for the great outbreaks of ancient 'plague' the two became one and have remained so. However, careful consideration of the accounts of the Black Death reveals certain features which are inconsistent with our modern knowledge of bubonic plague and its variants, the most obvious relating to the biology of the plague vectors. After considering these characteristics I came to have reservations about the causation of the Black Death. The analysis of all these matters forms the substance of this book.

We cannot take the medieval pandemic in isolation and it must be considered in relation to earlier plagues and related closely to more recent events. Thus I have also considered the evidence for the earlier plagues because some features recur in the Middle Ages and these may be important. The whole of the past plague record must naturally be set against our modern knowledge of plague gained in the past one hundred years with the modern techniques and approach to vector biology and I have used this information as the basic data with which past epidemics may be compared.

It is believed that there have been three plague pandemics. The first of these is said to have begun in A.D. 542, beginning in the fifteenth year of the reign of the Emperor Justinian. The second, the Black Death, spread across Europe in the years 1347–50 and came via the Crimean ports, lasting until 1720 when it finally left Europe. The third and current pandemic began during the second half of the nineteenth century and makes a good starting point to introduce the biology of plague.

The necessary components of plague are rodents (often rats), fleas and the bacillus which is the causative organism. A convenient point to begin the plague cycle is with a carrier species of rodent such as the rat. In the blood of this animal the bacillus *Yersinia pestis* multiplies rapidly and produces an overwhelming septicaemia. If fleas are present on the rat, a flea will take in a large number of bacteria in the blood meal and these pass into the flea's stomach. In about only twelve per cent of fleas the bacteria become established in the stomach and, by dividing rapidly, form a solid mass which fills it. Such a flea is known as a 'blocked' flea (Bacot & Martin, 1914) (Fig. 1), because no blood can enter the stomach. A flea in this condition also becomes very hungry and will feed on any warm-blooded animal it can find, including man. On a human host a blocked flea will suck blood until the gullet distends to its limit but eventually the elasticity of the gullet walls will cause it to contract and regurgitate some blood back into the wound. This blood has contacted and picked up plague bacilli which now enter the body of the host.

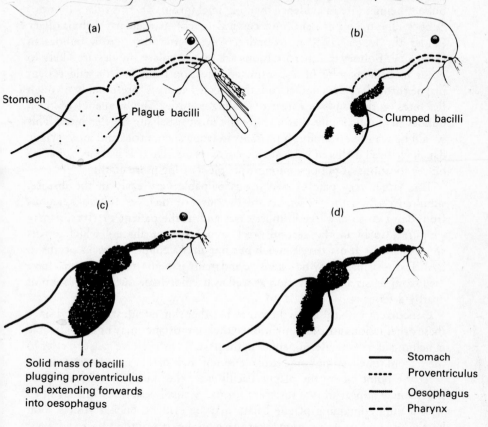

Fig. 1   Stages in the blocking of the flea proventriculus

As the flea feeds it automatically defaecates at the same time and deposits bacteria in the faeces. Scratching to relieve the irritation rubs the organisms into the puncture made by the mouth parts of the flea or into skin abrasions.

It is important to bear in mind that some members of a population of a rat species and some other rodent species too, actually die from a plague infection. When this happens the fleas leave the body of the dead animal as it cools and seek an alternative host in man or another mammal.

In typical human bubonic plague there is an incubation period of from two to eight days. At the end of this period, although bacilli may be present in the blood stream their numbers are small. They are chiefly concentrated in the lymph glands draining the extremities, that is those of the armpit, neck and groin. The lymph glands and their surrounding tissues swell and it is this swelling which is the primary bubo, the word 'bubo' being derived from the Greek word for groin. As a rule groin buboes are the most frequent, making up between 55 and 70 per cent of all recorded buboes with femoral (thigh) buboes being more in evidence than inguinal (groin) ones. Axillary (armpit) buboes, about 20 per cent, and cervical (neck), particularly submaxillary (under the lower jaw), at around ten per cent follow groin buboes in frequency. Buboes in other locations are rare. Axillary buboes are likely to occur in patients who have contracted infection from foci of wild rodent plague through direct contact with the affected animals (presumably through flea bites on the hands or forearm) (Pollitzer, 1954). The frequency of groin buboes may thus imply that legs are the most usual site for flea bites. This would be very likely amongst peasants in tropical countries and most plague data have been gathered from such environments. There is little information on the locations of buboes amongst people wearing more clothing.

This large, very painful swelling is palpable very early in the disease, simultaneously with, or even before, the onset of the fever. It is conspicuous from day two to day five in most cases and, if the patient survives, it may suppurate early in the second week and form an abscess which opens spontaneously. It discharges much pus but after a couple of weeks begins to heal. Tissue damage may be extensive and many patients in the past must have died from sepsis and exhaustion as well as haemorrhage due to ulceration of nearby arteries.

Concurrent with the bubo there may be other skin manifestations and since these other lesions are often mentioned their importance may be considerable in helping us to evaluate epidemics in the past. As I shall have cause to refer to them from time to time some explanation of their nature may be made here.

At the point where the plague bacilli enter the skin, primary cutaneous lesions may appear in two different forms. A small vesicle, or blister, filled with a fluid containing plague bacilli may be evident. Such a vesicle soon breaks and no further reaction takes place on the part of the adjacent tissues. Such lesions probably occur more often than they are recorded, probably because they are more frequent in benign than in grave cases of bubonic plague. Also at the site of infection carbuncles may develop. This process begins with the formation of ecchymotic or petechial spots[2] which increase in size. Primary plague carbuncles are usually small or of moderate size with a circumference rarely exceeding 2.5–5.0 cm. According to the site of infection they may form on different parts of the body and their appearance may coincide with, or precede, plague buboes. The prognosis is good when these marked reactions develop at the site of invasion.

As well as these lesions, secondary skin manifestations may develop in patients suffering from a severe form of the infection. These are skin haemorrhages which on some occasions are restricted to the vicinity of the bubo but may also appear on other parts of the body. If many petechiae or ecchymoses appear early in the disease it is an ominous sign (Pollitzer, 1954). According to this author marked skin manifestations have been rare in epidemics this century but seem to have been common during the Black Death and the London plague of 1665. It is believed that the words of the old nursery rhyme 'ring – a ring of roses' referred to the livid spots on the body, which were due to subcutaneous haemorrhages, when these occurred around the waist.

Despite these very obvious symptoms it is important to understand that none of these lesions, not even the bubo itself, is exclusive to plague and, as we shall see later, certain other criteria should be met before one accepts that a particular epidemic is indisputably bubonic plague.

Next to these local manifestations the most characteristic symptoms of plague are those which are associated with the nervous system. Simpson (1905) observed that the nervous reaction of patients to the toxin of the plague bacillus varied markedly. The most extreme cases might exhibit sudden transitions: 'patients who seem apathetic quite unexpectedly leaving their bed and trying to get into the open. Such restlessness is, on the whole, most often seen in the later stages of the disease, apparently because the patients then suffer "air hunger" '. There has been general agreement that plague produces a progressively intoxicating effect on the nervous system which displays itself with varying degrees of intensity in different ways on different constitutions. Some patients show insomnia, others a wild delirium and some stupor. In all is seen a loss of co-ordinating power over the voluntary muscles, coupled with a dulling of the senses.

In typical bubonic plague the disease is usually insidious in onset but rapid in progress. Occasionally, though, large numbers of the bacteria get into the blood stream and, without the localising and arresting effects of the axillary lymph nodes, the whole infection falls on the animal in a body-wide attack. An intense septicaemia occurs before death in fatal cases. In primary septicaemic plague the illness is short, so short that lymph nodes are not involved to any marked degree and most organisms are found in the spleen. It is very likely that reported cases from the past in which people retired to bed fit and died in the night were cases of septicaemic plague, the progression from vigorous health to prostration and death taking place in a few hours. Cases of septicaemic plague are infrequent and there is only a very short period when bacilli are in the blood but it is when this form of plague is in evidence that the human flea, *Pulex irritans*, may operate. The flea can take in large numbers of bacilli and carry the disease to a new host without the need of a rat to provide fresh sources of infection. In normal bubonic plague, however, even in the blood of fatal cases, bacilli are few and far between and the human flea would therefore be ineffective as a man to man transmitter since there would be insufficient bacilli to colonise the stomach of the flea. Bubonic plague scarcely ever spreads from man to man, even when fleas are plentiful, a point which is well worth emphasising and will be referred to again when considering the spread of medieval plague.

During normal bubonic plague, organisms may find their way into the lungs of the patient and there produce the third variant, pneumonic plague. The focus then exists in the lungs with a sudden, haemorrhagic bronchopneumonia. The bacteria are found in the bronchopneumonic areas and occur in the sputum of patients. This is infectious and the droplet-borne nature of this form of plague enables it to be spread without the intermediation of fleas. In epidemics of the late nineteenth century, when treatment was little different from that in the Middle Ages, 60 to 90 per cent of bubonic cases died. With the pneumonic form, the death rate if untreated is 100 per cent and in the Manchurian pneumonic epidemic of 1921 the average expectation of life was 1.8 days (Chun, 1936). The nursery rhyme previously referred to was completed with the line 'a-tishoo, a-tishoo, we all fall down', believed to be a reference to pneumonic plague. However, this form of plague rarely persists for long as an independent disease in the absence of the bubonic form. Of the three, bubonic is therefore the least infectious. The breath is not affected and the patient has died or recovered before enough bacilli have accumulated in the blood to make it infective for the flea. Cases of bubonic plague could be nursed in a general hospital.

Gill (1928) pointed out that an exceptional degree of complexity was added to the plague problem because primary pneumonic plague, bubonic plague, septicaemic plague and *pestis minor* were often regarded as distinctive diseases. Thus the quite distinctive clinical and epidemiological features shown by the various forms of plague might merely be dependent upon the site of selection, the route of invasion, the channel of infection or the mode of transmission of the parasite. Bubonic plague therefore could be regarded as representing the disease concept associated with invasion of the plague bacillus via the skin and lymphatics and *pestis minor* that shown by a small dose of infection or a high degree of resistance. Septicaemic plague signs resulted from the bacteria overwhelming the resistance of the lymphatic system and becoming established in a site favourable to their multiplication. In primary pneumonic plague, the entrance of the organism to the lungs via the respiratory tract enabled it to reach an environment peculiarly favourable to its proliferation, an assumption amply supported from the condition of the lungs after death and of the sputum in life.

The adult rodent flea (Fig. 2) lives upon warm-blooded animals such as birds or mammals. It is small (about 3 mm in length), wingless, adapted for clinging by means of hooks on its limbs, and it feeds only upon the host, taking blood with its piercing and sucking mouth parts which form a tube with a sharpened end.

When a plague-infected rodent dies of the disease and the fleas leave the corpse as the body temperature falls, some, not readily finding a new host,

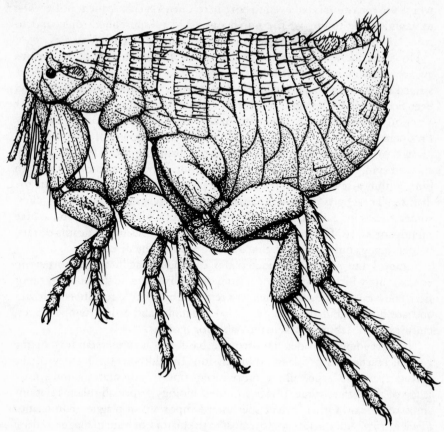

Fig. 2 Adult rat flea, *Xenopsylla cheopis* ♂ × 50 after Jordan and Rothschild and Imms

will be forced to remain on the ground, perhaps for some time. If temperature and humidity are optimal 'blocked' fleas may survive and remain infected for at least six weeks although they are probably not able to transmit plague effectively for more than fourteen days (Shrewsbury, 1971). Such infected fleas could travel in merchandise and, being very hungry, would immediately attack people unpacking the products. Within a short period of time those people would be ill with plague, but the few cases at this stage would be confined to those who had handled the goods. There would then, according to Shrewsbury, be a period of about two weeks during which time the freed 'blocked' fleas infected the local rats in the store or house. This would be followed by an epizootic (the rodent equivalent of a human epidemic) of rat-plague which would result in an increase in further 'blocked' fleas and the subsequent transmission of many infections to the human population bringing about a local epidemic of bubonic plague.

It is vital, in any analysis of alleged medieval or later plague outbreaks, where the causation is believed to have been due to such a sequence of events, to examine the timing of the initial cases and of subsequent ones and to compare the pattern with known twentieth-century plague epidemics.

However, there may be considerable variation in the timing of the various events following plague introduction as Simond (in Hankin, 1905) demonstrated in Western India. He showed that when the infectious material had been brought into a village it frequently did not manifest its activity until after a period of weeks or *even months*. According to Hankin, both in Bombay Presidency and in Garhwal the typical mode of development of an outbreak of known history was as follows: the person bringing the infection usually showed symptoms, together with a varying number of people in contact with him, within a few days and within the probable incubation period of the disease. There was then a quiescent period, generally of twenty days, sometimes as little as ten days and sometimes for a longer period up to three months or more. The first sign of renewed activity was in the deaths of rats, human beings only falling victim after rats died of the disease.

Some of the physical characteristics of plague bacilli are important in considering which conditions will keep them alive outside the body of rat or flea. They are killed by being held at a temperature of 55° c for fifteen minutes and are quickly killed when dried. If kept moist and at low temperatures, cultures in the laboratory remain viable for months.

The foregoing provides an adequate basis for an understanding of the general mechanism of plague transmission. In addition, the history of the spread of plague, especially in more recent times, necessitates some knowledge of the different rat species and their biology, especially their relationships with man. Other rodent species are important in plague maintenance (Twigg, 1978) but the rats are foremost in the history of human plague and are still the chief danger as plague transmitters to man in urban environments, their dead bodies giving the first indications that plague is present in a locality.

There are two main rat species, although very many sub-species and forms can also be identified. These two rats are the Brown rat, *Rattus norvegicus*, and the Black rat, *Rattus rattus*. The latter is a descendant of a rat which probably originated in India and spread along trading routes to establish itself as the common rat of both town and countryside in the tropics. Contrary to some authors, it is widely spread away from seaports in the tropics when there are no indigenous rodent competitors; in many places, especially islands, it is the common rat of the countryside. In temperate latitudes it is confined to buildings because for most of the year the outdoor temperatures are too low for its liking. Being a good climber it has readily gained access to ships which have transported it over much of the world. In buildings it climbs to the higher levels and lives in the roofs and ceilings rather than the basement. The Brown rat, on the other hand, is a less accomplished climber and inhabits the cellars and lower floors. This species spread from Russia in the early part of the eighteenth century and has since gone to most parts of the world. Being more hardy than the Black rat it is the common rat of temperate latitudes, living both in and out of doors. In the tropics it is confined mainly to ports and towns and lives close to human habitation in the countryside.

In evaluating plague in rodents two important phases can be distinguished. When the disease is confined to rats – as it usually is when being carried by ship or when it is present in the rats of a port – it is said to be in the 'murine' phase. Frequently it transfers from the rats to the endemic rodents such as gerbils or ground squirrels whose populations cover vast areas of country and it is then said to be in the 'sylvatic' phase (Twigg, 1978).

One point which should be borne in mind is the importance of the human role in the maintenance of the disease. In those disease organisms which depend upon man for their survival during its life cycle, there is either a process of decline in virulence of the disease organism or increased human resistance after the disease first makes its impact on a human population. For example, it is thought that syphilis and pulmonary tuberculosis have respectively conformed to these two alternatives. Bubonic plague, however, has no need of man who is merely an accidental or incidental host. It does depend, though, for its survival on the rodent and the flea and especially on a reservoir of resistant fleas and rodents. If both flea and rodent died then the disease itself would be exterminated.

As we have already seen, some rats in a population will be resistant to the disease so that despite the deaths of many the plague will exist enzootically in the murine population and become epizootic from time to time, causing human cases. Amongst rodents in the sylvatic phase a similar state of affairs is seen and whilst such plague epizootics in, for example, gerbils may be of less importance for man, nevertheless the disease may be passed to the local murine rodents who in turn will infect man.

It seems likely, as has been maintained by Wu, Lien-Teh (1936), that plague has been present since time immemorial in areas within or near the central Asiatic plateau and that this should be considered the home of the disease. During the first half of the nineteenth century plague became established in the west of Yun-nan, China, although it did not reach serious proportions. In 1855 a rebellion of Mohammedans began and in order to suppress them troops were sent to the area. As a probable consequence of these operations and the flight of the refugees, the plague spread. It moved steadily, reaching the provincial capital Yun-nan-fu (now Kunming) in 1866 and it was not until 1894, 28 years later, that it reached Canton and Hong Kong.

By this time the steamship was replacing sail, reducing the time at sea and carrying larger cargoes. The Chinese ports were some of the busiest and from the rat-infested warehouses plague was carried by rats and fleas to most parts of the world, some areas which had never before experienced plague becoming infected at this time. Others, such as India, parts of North and East Africa and the Mediterranean had had a history of plague, although at the time they were mainly plague-free. In these areas plague was soon active again.

The sub-continent of India was first infected via Calcutta in 1895 and through Bombay in 1896. Plague continued in Calcutta until 1925 with peak years from 1900 to 1907. After a plague-free spell of 23 years plague returned in 1948, with a peak year in 1949. In Bombay the disease was severe until 1923 when it waned, finally ceasing in 1935 although it was to reappear in 1948 and again in 1949 and 1952.

The Indian experience illustrates very well the part played by rats in human plague outbreaks and later, in the analysis of medieval outbreaks, comparisons will be made with Indian conditions which in many ways are the closest parallel to those in fourteenth-century Europe. In the major Indian cities the proportions of the two rat species have varied. In Madras *Rattus rattus* was dominant until 1930 when it was almost the only species. In Calcutta the same rat made up only 14.0 per cent of the rodent species in 1906 and stayed at that level until 1950. Since the epidemic of 1948–52 its percentage has been reduced by half. The Brown rat has not been strongly represented in Calcutta and has fluctuated between 9.0 and 26.0 per cent in the few years preceding 1960 (Seal, 1969a).

In Bombay, between 1910 and 1956, the proportions of *Rattus rattus* and *Rattus norvegicus* changed markedly: in 1910 *R. rattus* made up 66 per cent of rodents but by 1956 only 23–24 per cent. Similarly, the proportions of *Rattus norvegicus* changed, from 29 per cent in 1910 to 16 per cent in 1956. The reason for this has been that the rodent *Bandicota bengalensis* has increased its numbers considerably and in 1960 comprised between 49 and 50 per cent of the rodents, whereas in 1910 it made up only one per cent. This species is fairly susceptible to plague but *Rattus rattus* and *Rattus norvegicus* were both still very resistant in 1960.

A proportion of rats in a population succumbs to plague and the following shows how species resistance to plague bacilli may vary:

Percentage mortality among Bombay rats in resistance tests

	1952	1953	1954	1955	1956
R. rattus	12.6	13.7	12.1	10.0	7.5
R. norvegicus	—	5.8	3.3	2.6	2.2
B. bengalensis	77.6	82.5	76.7	70.0	75.2

The mortality figures for rodents in Calcutta in 1953–54 were rather different, however:

R. rattus	31.0 per cent
R. norvegicus	94.7 per cent
B. bengalensis	97.6 per cent

Yet in Madras both species of *Rattus* were fully susceptible.

This question of rodent resistance, either of species or of individuals within a species, is clearly of great importance in plague epidemiology. What is equally important is the flea species carried by the rodents and whilst I propose to deal with this more fully later it is of importance in the Indian context to draw attention to the matter.

The flea species *Xenopsylla cheopis* has a close association with rats and is an efficient flea from the point of plague transmission. From early this century up to 1960 the data from India indicate that *Rattus rattus* among rodents and *X. cheopis* among fleas are the two most important elements in urban human plague infection, the role of *Rattus norvegicus* being a lesser one. It is of interest that Madras, with a reputation of being almost entirely plague-free, had only 5.6 per cent of *X. cheopis* in its flea total in 1931, 94.3 per cent consisting of *X. astia*.

In India between 1898 and 1957, 12,707,475 people died of plague (Seal, 1969b). The success of plague in India was aided by overcrowding of people and a climate favourable to rats and fleas. Because of the severity of the Indian situation the Indian Plague Commission came into being to study the disease and its carriers. Certain features of plague epidemics had been known long before this and epidemiologists and medical practitioners in China had long since associated rat plague with human plague. The inhabitants of Garhwal, Uganda and Yun-nan are said to have evacuated villages at the first evidence of rat mortality as a precaution. I say 'are said to have' because the reporting of so many features of plague, this one included, has not been as accurate as one would wish and there has been a tendency to select features supporting plague and its folklore when the actual story is less straightforward and perhaps open to other interpretation. The following paragraph from Bannerman (1906) is a case in point. He said:

> In India from the earliest times of which any record exists it appears to have been the habit to desert the infected towns or villages on the appearance of plague, and this practice continues to the present day in the endemic focus of Kumaon in the Himalayas. On the appearance of plague in Kumaon the people of their own accord evacuate the village; and erecting for themselves huts in the jungle, live there for some months till they consider it safe to return.

This information he ascribed to Hutcheson (1895). However, the account by Hutcheson says that whilst there was mention of rat deaths preceding human illness in an outbreak in May, 1888, this mahamari was called 'hill plague, or a severe type of typhus fever highly contagious and bred and fostered by filth'. He points out that the history of the disease is imperfect owing to confusion arising from adopting the view that mahamari and sanjar, or typhus fever, were identical diseases. The reports of various doctors who had been involved in epidemics in the area were quoted by Hutcheson, for example:

> Dr Richardson reported that typhus fever, identical with mahamari, prevailed more or less throughout the year 1884 in the Kumaon Division.

Dr Renny, on 9 May 1850 commenced a local investigation. He described the disease as an infectious fever of a malignant kind and of a typhus character, accompanied by glandular tumours.

Dr Thomson reported on the outbreak of mahamari, identical with typhus fever in April and May 1886.

There appears, therefore, to be some doubt about the true identity of *mahamari*, but there was rodent mortality as already seen, and again in 1876 when:

the inhabitants of Barkuri vacated their village on the 22nd July, 1876, on account of a great mortality among rats and mice, and an outbreak of mahamari was thus in all probability averted. At first the sick were nursed and died in the houses, afterwards the sick were nursed and died in temporary huts outside the village.

In another outbreak in 1876–7, after 13 deaths:

the people of the villages vacated their houses so soon as gola or bubo was noticed as a symptom of the diseases in those who lived beyond the fifth day. Indeed, deaths from gola being reported, the civil authorities directed the people to vacate their houses and they located themselves in huts of grass and branches on the hillside.

Hutcheson makes no mention of this being the practice from earliest times. He surmises that *mahamari* and plague are the same disease 'which has existed in all probability in the hill tracts of India and China from time immemorial'. It is unfortunate that more clinical detail is not available in this account so that a better picture of the actual diseases involved could be seen. In addition, it would have been of great value to have had some idea of what the rats and mice were dying from and whether they lived in the houses or in the fields. There may have been plague and perhaps other diseases as well. The point I wish to emphasise is that Bannerman has taken the term plague out of its context of hill plague and used it synonymously with bubonic plague, ignored the other disease, or diseases, present and extended the evacuation of villages from the recorded recent events to the far distant past.

Long before the Plague Research Commission reported in 1908, the relation between fatal rodent plague and human epidemics was recognised. During the late eighteenth century Shih Tao-nan, a native of Chaochow, China, wrote a poem called 'Death of rats', part of which read:

Dead rats in the east,
Dead rats in the west.

As if they were tigers,
Indeed are the people afraid.

Few days following the death of rats,
Men pass away like falling walls.

Then comes a stanza which casts some doubt on the nature of the disease because, if accurate, it does not fit any of the manifestations of plague:

While three men are walking together
Two drop dead within ten steps.

The author of this poem died of plague almost immediately after completing it (Wu, Lien-Teh, 1936).

Indian natives long recognised that some connection existed between rats and plague in the saying: 'When the rats begin to fall it is time for people to leave the houses', i.e. a plague outbreak was preceded by rat mortality.

In the early years of the present pandemic the importance of the association of rat plague and human plague became clear to workers in China, India, Formosa and Australia. The relationship between the epizootic and the epidemic was clearly brought out in Australia by Thompson (1900, 1906) and by Tidswell (1900). On account of the relatively small size of the outbreak and the fact that it involved an entirely European population, a detailed investigation of each case was accomplished. From these observations Thompson concluded:

1. that plague in rats preceded the first case which occurred in man;
2. the epizootic area was co-extensive with the epidemic area;
3. the epidemic was due to communication of infection from rat to man.

These findings have been shown to be of central importance in any plague outbreak and must be kept in mind when examining the nature of medieval epidemics.

From the southern China focus plague was transported to South Africa, where it had never been before. Between 1899 and 1903 the disease occurred in all the main South African ports and epidemics broke out, the most severe being those at Cape Town with 766 cases of which 371 were fatal, and Durban with 145 fatalities from 201 cases. The murine phase lasted until 1912 and soon afterwards it was suspected that the sylvatic phase was beginning because in 1914–15 a series of plague outbreaks occurred on farms in remote rural areas in the Cape Midlands. It was suspected that these had their origin in wild rodents but it was not until 1921 that this was proved (Mitchell, 1927).

East Africa is believed to have been affected by plague in the sixth century A.D. (Roberts, 1935) and there is a record of plague in this region at Mombasa in 1697 during a siege of Portuguese by the Arabs which lasted almost three years. Plague, if such it was, probably spread from the caravan routes from the north to the east coast and it was known in the north-eastern Congo by the Ituri people and at Kisumu on Lake Victoria. Throughout the eighteenth and nineteenth centuries epidemics alleged to be plague occurred at Kisumu in Kenya and during the last three decades of the nineteenth century, and especially from 1880 onwards, there are records of outbreaks from a variety of localities around Lake Victoria, central Tanzania and at a few localities in southern and south-eastern Kenya.

At the beginning of the twentieth century oriental plague appeared in East African ports from India and at the same time some of the old foci in East Africa were reactivated. The bacillus of *Yersinia pestis* was identified at Kisiba on the western side of Lake Victoria by Robert Koch and Kupitza in 1897. Human activities, especially migration and transport have contributed largely to plague spread: the construction of the Uganda railway from Mombasa to Kisumu between 1896 and 1901 assisted the spread of plague. In 1905 a railway line was begun from Dar-es-Salaam to Lake Tanganyika which it reached in 1914. This line also closely followed the original trade routes along which, presumably, the earliest spread took place and in so doing linked up several of the dormant plague foci.

Egypt had been free of plague for 55 years but in 1899 it re-appeared at Alexandria, in 1900 at Port Said and in 1904 at Suez, moving inland from these centres of introduction and reaching most parts of the Nile Valley to Aswan. Plague re-appeared in Tunis in 1907 after being absent from the coastal areas of North Africa west of Egypt since 1822.

Between 1895 and 1903 most of the major ports in the tropics became plague infected; in many cases the disease transferred before long to the sylvatic phase and became widespread across the continents. Especially

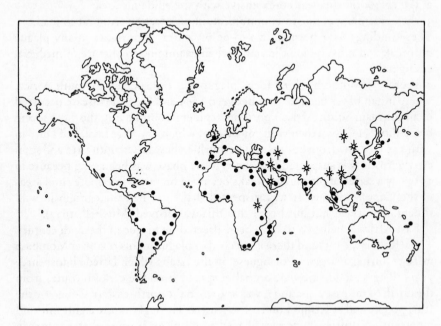

Fig. 3 Ancient plague foci (starred) and the spread of plague during the late nineteenth and early twentieth centuries (solid black dots)

striking in this respect was the spread in southern Africa and across North America. Figure 3 shows those localities where long-standing plague foci of ancient origin still existed and all the localities which became infected from 1894 onwards.

Finally, one very important point must be made about this pandemic. Although plague was being successfully introduced, or re-introduced, to many parts of the world it is significant that, with one exception which will be discussed later, it did not invade Europe. It is true that there were isolated cases of bubonic plague in several ports and infected rats were on occasion recovered, but there was little rat to rat spread and no sylvatic phase. This single fact is of great importance in the analysis of disease outbreaks in Europe in the fourteenth century.

CHAPTER TWO

Plague before A.D. *1348*

The word plague is derived from the Latin *plaga*, meaning a blow or a stroke, but in medieval Latin (Latham, 1965) it came to mean a plague or a pestilence. With the sense of 'epidemic' or 'disastrous abundance, of an animal species the word has apparently been used in English for a long time, but as a word referring to a specific bacterial disease, said to be bubonic plague, it was not used until the seventeenth century (Shrewsbury, 1971). Therefore, the term plague, when used earlier than this in English accounts or in translations from Greek or Latin, cannot be accepted as referring specifically to bubonic plague unless there is clear confirmatory evidence. Shrewsbury makes quite clear that the evidence that is required to identify a pestilence in the distant past as an epidemic of bubonic plague may be either a contemporary description of the clinical picture of the disease that is characteristic of plague or a combination of certain observations that are exclusive to the epidemiology of plague. Unless one, and preferably both of these conditions are fulfilled, he considers that the assumption that an ancient pestilence was an epidemic of bubonic plague is not justifiable.

The problem of assessing the true nature of past epidemics is a difficult one. Writers in the distant past have left us accounts of some of the more obvious physical symptoms of plague and of other diseases also. Unfortunately, more than one disease may produce the same symptoms; this, coupled with the sketchiness of contemporary accounts, especially in Britain, has resulted in very little for the modern worker to assess. Shrewsbury, in advice on the identification of past epidemics, emphasised this when he pointed out that the bubo and other skin manifestations of the bubonic form, and the bloody sputum of pneumonic plague, together with the experience that recovery from an attack of the disease did not confer immunity against subsequent attacks, comprised all that was known about plague in the British Isles up to the end of the seventeenth century and was all that the historian could expect to obtain from contemporary accounts of epidemics of the disease. Furthermore, when contemporary accounts of ancient diseases do not give adequate information for them to be identified as plague, then any scholar attempting to identify a pestilence as plague has to show that the house rat was established in the society at that time.

These rigorous criteria must be applied to early epidemics or pandemics along with an analysis of other factors if we are to determine the presence of true plague. The major part of this thesis will be devoted to the outbreaks of the fourteenth century but earlier outbreaks will also be considered. In some cases descriptions from early times are much more helpful than are those from the fourteenth century A.D. and we can be more certain that the pestilence referred to was bubonic plague.

Many past epidemics have been claimed to be bubonic plague. One biblical outbreak, the plague of the Philistines, is generally believed to be so but in a detailed analysis of the symptoms and supporting information Shrewsbury (1964) came to the conclusion that this particular disease outbreak was probably dysentery.

The epidemic which broke out at Athens in 430 B.C. has often been said to be bubonic plague. Thucydides, in his account of the Peloponnesian War, described how this pestilence broke out in the summer and described the symptoms at some length:

> Many who were in perfect health, all in a moment, and without any apparent reason, were seized with violent heats in the head and with redness and inflammation of the eyes. Internally the throat and the tongue were quickly suffused with blood, and the breath became unnatural and fetid. There followed sneezing and hoarseness; in a short time the disorder, accompanied by a violent cough, reached the chest; then fastening lower down it would move the stomach and bring on all the vomits of bile to which physicians have ever given names; and they were very distressing. An inefficient retching producing violent convulsions attacked most of the sufferers; some as soon as the previous symptoms had abated, others not until long afterwards. The body externally was not so very hot to the touch, nor yet pale; it was of a livid colour inclining to red, and breaking out in pustules and ulcers. But the internal fever was intense; the sufferers could not bear to have on them even the finest linen garment; they insisted on being naked, and there was nothing which they longed for more eagerly than to throw themselves into cold water. And many of those who had no one to look after them actually plunged into the cisterns, for they were tormented by increasing thirst, which was not in the least assuaged whether they drank little or much.
>
> They could not sleep; a restlessness which was intolerable never left them. While the disease was at its height the body, instead of wasting away, held out amid these sufferings in a marvellous manner, and either they died on the seventh or ninth day, not of weakness, for their strength was not exhausted, but of internal fever, which was the end of most; or if they survived, then the disease descended into the bowels and there produced violent ulceration; severe diarrhoea at the same time set in, and at a later stage caused exhaustion, which

finally with few exceptions carried them off. For the disorder which had originally settled in the head passed gradually through the whole body, and, if a person got over the worst, would often seize the extremities and leave its mark, attacking the privy parts and the fingers and the toes; and some escaped with the loss of these, some with the loss of their eyes. Some again had no sooner recovered than they were seized with a forgetfulness of all things and knew neither themselves nor their friends.

He goes on to comment upon one circumstance in particular which distinguished this malady from ordinary diseases. Although there were so many bodies lying unburied, the birds and animals which normally fed on human flesh either never came near them or died if they touched them. This was, he said, proved by a remarkable disappearance of the birds of prey, who were not to be seen either about the bodies or anywhere else, and in the case of the dogs the fact was even more obvious because they lived with man.

It would be interesting to know how accurate was the observation concerning the death of animals which had fed upon human flesh. It could be relevant in certain diseases but not where bubonic plague was the cause of death. On no occasion does Thucydides draw attention to buboes, a fact which is remarkable if it was bubonic plague because of the obvious nature of these swellings. The symptoms resemble a combination of influenza and a gastric infection and the disease was said to have begun in Ethiopia, from where it moved to Egypt, Libya, the greater part of the Persian empire and then Athens. It seems very unlikely that this was bubonic plague and Macarthur (1959) has presented a detailed examination of the outbreak which he was in no doubt was typhus fever.

One of the early and most detailed accounts of plague is that of Procopius in the history of the Persian Wars. He wrote that during those times (A.D. 542) there was a pestilence by which the whole human race came near to being annihilated and that the plague attacked some in the summer season, others in the winter, and still others at the other times of the year. It is unlikely, from modern knowledge, that bubonic plague was responsible for illness in all the seasons of the year. Procopius claimed that the plague started from the Egyptians who dwelt in Pelusium. Then it divided and moved in one direction towards Alexandria and the rest of Egypt, and in the other direction it came to Palestine 'and from there it spread over the whole world, always moving forward and travelling at times favourable to it'.

He points out that the disease always began at the coast and from there went to the interior. Both plague and any other infectious disease might behave in this way for all new arrivals from any distance away were most likely to come by sea and hence start the infection in a port. If we knew the speed at which the plague spread it would help us assess what type of epidemic disease was in operation.

Procopius presents a mixture of information: on the one hand he gives details of the symptoms which encourage us to have enough confidence in his accounts to say that bubonic plague was present whilst on the other hand he mixes in quaint superstition, the presentation of which tends to make us cautious about the descriptions of physical symptoms. For example, speaking of how people became ill he says that apparitions of supernatural beings in human guise of every description were seen by many persons, and those who encountered them thought that they were struck by the man they had met in one or other part of the body and immediately upon seeing this apparition they were seized also by the disease.

On the subject of physical symptoms, he describes the onset of a sudden fever which was of such a languid sort that neither the sick nor the physician was suspicious of danger. Then on the same day in some cases, in others on the following day, and in the rest a few days later, a bubonic swelling developed; this took place not only in the groin but also inside the armpit, and in some cases also behind the ears, and at different points on the thighs.

Up to this point all who had the disease appeared to be much the same, but from then on marked differences developed. Some went into a deep coma whilst others became violently delirious, yet in either case they suffered the characteristic symptoms of the disease. Many of the patients became frenzied and rushed to water whilst others could not easily take food.

In some cases death came immediately, in others after many days and with some the body broke out with black pustules about as large as a lentil and these did not survive even one day, but all succumbed immediately. With many also a vomiting of blood occurred without visible cause and these people died straight away. Physicians who opened buboes in the dead found a strange sort of carbuncle that had grown inside them. In cases where the bubo became very large and burst, discharging pus, the patients survived. Clearly, there is much in this account that leads us to think that bubonic plague was present although there may also have been other diseases.

As to the mortality estimations, however, the figures must surely be greatly exaggerated. The disease in Constantinople lasted for four months and its greatest virulence for three. Procopius states that at first the deaths were a little more than the normal, then the mortality rose until it reached 5,000 each day, later becoming 10,000 and still more than that. At a rough estimate, using the type of mortality curve seen in London in the summer of 1665 or in India in the early part of the twentieth century, the number of dead must have been round about 600,000. By contrast the number of alleged plague deaths in London in 1665 for the whole year was 68,596. The total population at that time is generally agreed to have been about 400,000, the plague therefore killing 17.15 per cent of the population. If the same sort of relationship held for Constantinople in A.D. 542 the total population could have been almost 3,500,000. This seems too high and if we bear in mind that the mortality in Britain in 1348–9 during the Black Death was held to be around one-third of the population then the total population of Constantinople would be nearer

1,800,000. In fact it is most unlikely that it was anything like as high as this. Russell (1968) considered that the city did not have more than 300,000 people so either estimates of the dead were grossly exaggerated or else there was an abnormally high mortality.

Beginning in A.D. 540 in the Roman Empire in the east was a major epidemic of which the outbreak in Constantinople recorded by Procopius in A.D. 542 was a part. This is known as the plague of Justinian. According to Russell (1968) this plague continued as a series of epidemics well into the seventh century and followed a pattern similar to that of the fourteenth-century Black Death. The Byzantine Emperor Justinian had previously recaptured North Africa from the Vandals and much of Italy from the Ostrogoths and there was every prospect of re-establishing the whole Roman Empire. Russell claims that the plague reduced the population by 40 to 50 per cent by the end of the sixth century and as a result of this high mortality and the reduction of the field armies, Islam took Egypt and Syria and extended its hold in the nomadic and semi-nomadic areas.

There is agreement that bubonic plague was present but Shrewsbury (1971) has pointed out that during this period certain other serious diseases were almost certainly evident. These were smallpox, probably diphtheria, either cholera or bacillary dysentery and also epidemic influenza. Any one of these, especially if appearing in a human population for the first time, would have a dramatic effect and could produce a death rate equal to, or even exceeding, that due to bubonic plague. If, as seems certain from Procopius, bubonic plague was there simultaneously with any one or more of the others, then a heavy toll of human life could be expected.

For bubonic plague to exist over a wide area for any length of time there must be an extensive population of a rodent species receptive to plague and harbouring fleas in which plague bacilli can grow. Unless such a rodent exists, plague fleas brought in by merchandise will cause little more than a few localised cases. The rodent in this case would almost certainly have been the Black or ship rat which is thought to have spread westwards from India before the Christian era, although exactly when is not clear. Shrewsbury (1971) asserts that the certain history of plague begins somewhere in the lands bordering on the eastern end of the Mediterranean, some time between 300 B.C. and the beginning of Christianity. As he points out, the nature of plague demands that whenever it appears it must be preceded by an intensive colonisation by the rat. He thinks that the trade which the Roman Empire developed with India was the key feature in the colonisation of the area. Whether this is so or not is difficult to say, but the unequivocal presence of extensive plague would be clear evidence that rats were present.

The Black rat is a species which shows no great liking for the cold. Its home area India has, over most of the sub-continent, temperatures favourable to this rat all the year round. When it moved to the west and occupied the Near East and the Mediterranean coastlands, it moved to a climatic zone where winters were cold enough to limit its outdoor living and make it dependent upon human habitation for warmth and shelter. Even in India the Black rat shows a preference for living in dwellings and is commonly called the house rat in the literature. Around the Mediterranean and in southern Europe the Black rat is today mainly a house rat and shows none of the tendency to live permanently out of doors away from man that the Brown rat does.

During the sixth century A.D. sea trading was flourishing in the Mediterranean and certain ports such as Marseilles were becoming very important. Pirenne (1939) considers that the population of Marseilles must have become large because of the many outbreaks of disease epidemics that took place between 566 and 591. Ships were regularly carrying cargoes from Alexandria and the Levant along the shores of Italy and Provence to Marseilles. The rat must have been well distributed around the Mediterranean and there are reports of epidemics of plague in the province of Arles (southern France) in 547, at Constantinople in 558, Italy 591, Liguria (the coastal state in which lies Genoa) in 566 and of five epidemics in southern France and northern Italy between 566 and 600. If these were all bubonic plague, and according to Shrewsbury they were, then the rat was probably well established.

Gregory of Tours observed the manner in which plague spread in the city of Marseilles:

> A ship had put into the port with the usual merchandise from Spain, unhappily bringing the timber which kindled this disease. Many citizens purchased various objects from the cargo, and soon a house inhabited by eight people was left empty, every one of them being carried off by the contagion. The fire of this plague did not spread immediately through all the houses in the place; but there was a certain interval, and then the whole city blazed with the pest, like a cornfield set aflame.

People presumably left the city for he says:

> After two months the affliction ceased and the people returned, thinking the danger overpast. But the plague began once more, and all who had returned perished. On several other occasions Marseilles was afflicted by this death.

The interesting observation by Gregory, that plague did not spread at once when introduced into a town (as a disease which spread directly from man to man would do), could reflect the period when the epizootic was spreading among the rats of the town. As rats died 'blocked' fleas no longer had hosts and then attacked men and the human epidemic was under way. The phrase used by Gregory that 'the whole city blazed with the pest, like a cornfield set aflame', is a remark which Shrewsbury considers to be an acute observation. Yet, as we shall see later, the history of plague introductions into even the large Indian cities with perhaps even greater crowding, more rats and a more favourable climate for flea breeding, has not produced epidemics that flared in that way. It is important that we know what sort of time interval Gregory was referring to if we are to draw effective biological deductions from the past epidemics. Unfortunately, this detail is lacking and despite the assumptions that have been made it does not seem to be an unequivocal guarantee that the disease was bubonic plague. It is true that some of what Gregory describes could be due to plague but there are other possibilities.

It is nevertheless worth repeating the exact words used by Bishop Gregory about the epidemic. About its effect on people and when it began he says, 'When, as I have above related, the blessed Quintianus had passed from this world, the holy Gall, with the kings' support, was appointed in his place. In his time raged the pestilence known as the plague of the groin in divers regions, but especially in the province of Arles'. He goes on to speak of its speed of action, 'For death came suddenly. There appeared in the groin or armpit a wound like that from a snakebite, and those who had it were swiftly destroyed by the poison, that on the second or third day they breathed their last.'

However, the plague of the groin occurred at the same time as other severe diseases, as the following shows: 'A great pestilence raged among the people during this year; great numbers were carried off by various malignant diseases, the symptoms of which were pustules and tumours; but many, by taking precautions, escaped. We heard in this year also of a malady of the groin which raged fiercely at Narbonne; it was of such a kind that if a man was once attacked, all was over with him.'

Speaking of plague elsewhere he refers to an epidemic in Rome in the fourteenth year of Kind Childebert; this was a pestilence called, 'the plague of the groin', apparently occurring in the middle of the eleventh month. These references to the groin have generally been construed as evidence of bubonic plague and, whilst not denying the possibility, it must be pointed out that buboes may occur in other bacterial and viral diseases, notably anthrax and smallpox. Nevertheless, they are more regularly present in bubonic plague than in any other disease.

In the year A.D. 590 the plague, 'Lues inguinaria', ravaged the cities of Viviers and Avignon according to Gregory and in April, A.D. 591, 'a terrible pestilence destroyed the people in the territory of Tours and in that of Nantes, the attack in each case being followed by a slight headache, soon after which the patient died'. There is little enough information here to make any opinion on what the ailment was. The death toll was reputedly high and in A.D. 571 Gregory records that there was such slaughter of the people that the legions of men who fell there could not be numbered. Normal burial practices broke down and when coffins and planks failed, ten dead or more were buried in a common pit. In one church on a certain Sunday 300 corpses were counted.

The Near East was an area of great importance at the time of Justinian. Traders were travelling both East and West, maritime commerce was brisk and all these movements of traders and armies must have brought a variety of epidemic diseases to the region. It is very probable that several other serious diseases in addition to bubonic plague were present and flaring up from time to time. Shrewsbury considers there is evidence of diphtheria, either bacillary dysentery or cholera and epidemic influenza. Indeed, as McNeill (1977) has suggested, the benefits of travel and trade with new regions may be to some extent offset by the acquisition of new diseases, either on the part of the travellers or, as in the case of the Spanish conquest of Mexico, on the part of the native inhabitants.

McNeill points out that the historical evidence suggests that the plagues of the sixth and seventh centuries were as important for Mediterranean peoples as was the more famous Black Death of the fourteenth century. He says that the disease certainly killed a large proportion of urban dwellers and that the reduced population took centuries to be restored. It would be valuable to have some actual statistics to support this but McNeill, pointing out the impossibility of precision, quotes only from Procopius on the death rates in Constantinople and I have commented earlier on those estimates. In the case of plague the distribution of the Black rat would certainly ensure that urban populations were most affected, and the same would be true for several other of the diseases mentioned by Shrewsbury. Corroborative evidence for the presence of other infectious diseases comes from the accounts by Muslim scholars of the destruction of the Abyssinian army which was attacking Mecca in the year A.D. 570. They suggested that the expedition was afflicted by smallpox and Ibn Ishag, an early biographer of the Prophet, reported that this was the first appearance of measles and smallpox among the Arabs (in Dols, 1974). Dols goes on to say:

> The possibility of a smallpox epidemic is given additional weight by the fact that the plague epidemics which struck Europe in the late sixth century coincided with violent epidemics of smallpox. It appears that the first serious epidemic of smallpox attacked most of continental Europe about the year 570. Yet we cannot be certain that the pestilence was smallpox, for the historical evidence is ambiguous and the vesicular form of plague may simulate smallpox; the pustules contain plague bacilli and this form of plague is highly fatal.

If he means the primary vesicles at the place where the bacilli enter the skin, the evidence is contrary to what Dols says and the prognosis is good.

None of the lesions, however, not even the bubo, is exclusive to plague and, according to Shrewsbury (1971), buboes may be present in cases of confluent smallpox. Russell (1968) also assumes that the bubo distinguishes plague from smallpox.

Historians have examined the consequences arising from the heavy mortality in the Mediterranean and Near East. Foremost among their conclusions is the belief that the failure of the Emperor Justinian to restore imperial unity to the Mediterranean is in some measure due to the effect plague had on the manpower of his forces. Also, the series of epidemics bringing heavy death tolls to the Mediterranean coastlands from 542 onwards is thought to have been the reason why Persian and Roman forces could only offer token resistance to the Moslem armies that swept out of Arabia in 634 (McNeill, 1977).

In a wider context, the long series of plagues which were confined almost entirely to territories within easy reach of Mediterranean ports have been thought by McNeill to have been part of the reason for the shift away from the Mediterranean as the centre of European civilisation and the increase in the importance of the lands to the north. Pirenne (1939) concluded that the advance of Islam separated East from West and that for the first time in history the axis of European life was shifted northwards from the Mediterranean but he never claimed that plague had any role in this change. Pirenne's ideas have, however, been challenged by Bautier (1971).

It seems likely that bubonic plague was present in some of the epidemics in the sixth century A.D. in lands around the Mediterranean, probably in association with other diseases whose impact have been equally severe and whose differentiation from bubonic plague was not easy to define at the time. On some occasions plague probably existed alone. Where it came from is even less clear: McNeill considers that it may have come from an old focus in north-east India or in central Africa and we know that of the three old foci of importance one of these was in the foothills of the Himalayas between India and China and the other was in central Africa in the region of the Great Lakes.

Pollitzer (1954) considered that the first really satisfactory evidence of bubonic plague was the pandemic beginning in A.D. 542 and believed that it came from Ethiopia, suggesting a central African origin. The Athens epidemic of 430 B.C. was also said to come from Ethiopia.

Plague disappeared from southern Europe towards the end of the sixth century and 700 years were to elapse before it returned. We presume that in order to sustain the epidemics around the Mediterranean there were Black rats at least in the ports and major cities. Shrewsbury states that, as late as the time of Justinian, the Black rat had probably not reached northern Europe. As a result of this, plague was confined to the Mediterranean coastlands within relatively easy reach of navigation. When, and how far north the Black rat moved is still not clear and will be discussed at some length later. Meanwhile, the position of northern Europe, especially the British Isles, will be examined *vis-à-vis* plague.

Britain A.D. 600–A.D. 1348

It appears highly improbable that there were any outbreaks of true plague in Europe during this period, although throughout Anglo-Saxon times there were epidemics called 'plague'. It is especially strange that the Mediterranean was free because plague had been widespread and rats were presumably permanent in towns. According to Shrewsbury (1971) the account by Pirenne (1939) and other historians of the growing Saracen empire which came to lie between Europe and India provides a convincing explanation for this lack of plague. It was assumed that bubonic plague had its homeland in India and was transmitted along the permanent chain of *Rattus rattus* which had been carried earlier to the Mediterranean. The interposition of the Saracen empire is thought to have interrupted the transfer of plague bacilli from East to West and, although epidemics of bubonic plague occurred in Mesopotamia and Asia Minor during this period, the bacilli were prevented from spreading westwards by the disruption of commerce that had brought plague into Europe in the sixth century.

Much has been written about the epidemics and 'plagues' which occurred in the British Isles in the Anglo-Saxon period and it is necessary to assess the medical evidence and decide which, if any, of these were bubonic plague.

It has been suggested that because Britain was an island it enjoyed greater immunity from plagues than did the rest of Europe. It is also said that during the later Middle Ages the roads of Britain, unlike those of the Continent, were not so much used by mercenaries or pilgrims, both of whom might carry disease from one region to another and that until the Norsemen came the British people were not subjected to invasions by people who would have brought new disease with them. None of these assertions are easy to substantiate or deny in a quantitative way. If true, then the British people might have had less disease from outside but on the other hand there would have been little chance to built up population resistance and so, when eventually the diseases arrived, the mortality would have been likely to be high, as it usually is when any infection reaches people lacking previous exposure to it. However, there is evidence that Anglo-Saxon trade with the Continent was considerable and it seems improbable that the British Isles could have been as isolated as suggested; disease may arrive by trading ships as easily as in warships.

There was no shortage of outbreaks of epidemics during Anglo-Saxon times between the years 526 and 1087 (Bonser, 1944). In addition, presumably worsening the effects of infectious organisms on the people, were the outbreaks of 'murrain' (infectious cattle disease) which killed many of the animals needed for food. Famines are also recorded during the period, on some occasions occurring during the same year that pestilence was present, so there was ample opportunity for disease to attack people already weakened by shortage of food.

Shrewsbury asserts strongly that it is clear that the house rat was settled in England in time to sustain the bubonic plague of the fourteenth century but that no pestilence occurring before that date can be identified as plague. Thus the 'pestis flava' which was rife in England in the sixth century could not have been bubonic plague. It clearly was severe and the mortality was by all accounts high, even allowing for the customary exaggeration. It was known as the Yellow Plague and several references bring this out: for the year A.D. 555 in the *Annals of Ulster* the *crón-conaill* (i.e. the *buidhe-conaill*), caused great mortality. Since *crón* means saffron and *buidhe* means yellow, this disease may have been some form of jaundice (Bonser, 1944).

In 550 the Yellow Plague was said to be roaming through the land in the guise of a loathly monster (Lloyd, 1939). This was in Wales but in Ireland too the plague was regarded as a living thing which roamed the land. The power of prayer against this creature was amply demonstrated when, at the prayer of St MacCreiche in Kerry, a fiery bolt from heaven fell upon it and reduced it to dust and ashes in the presence of the people.

This plague appeared again in the seventh century in A.D. 664 and outbreaks continued for many years. There are many records of this, more details than for any other plague of the Anglo-Saxon period. The *Anglo-Saxon Chronicle* (Garmonsway, 1955) refers to a great pestilence in 664. Bede, says, 'After this [i.e. May] in the same year there also suddenly arose a plague and sickness, which wasted and destroyed first the southern districts of Britain; but it also afflicted the province of Northumbria, and with fearful mortality long raged far and wide, killing and destroying a great multitude of men'. He also says, 'Ireland, the island of the Scots, was also assailed and ravaged with the same mortality'. This account has been taken to indicate that the disease was perhaps introduced into southern Britain, possibly from the Continent, and later spread northwards. It may simply, as Bede says, have arisen first in the south and later affected other areas. There is too little evidence either way to be certain how it arose.

This plague was apparently active during the summer months and the epidemic increased in violence in its second year. It is probably this plague which was described by Geoffrey of Monmouth (Thorpe, 1966):

> When Cadwallader fell ill, as I had begun to tell you, the Britons started to quarrel among themselves and to destroy the economy of their homeland by an appalling civil war. There then followed a second disaster: for a grievous and long-remembered famine afflicted the besotted population, and the countryside no longer produced any food at all for human sustenance, always excepting what the huntsman's skill could provide. A pestilent and deadly plague followed this famine and killed off such a vast number of the population that the living could not bury them. The few wretches left alive gathered themselves into bands and emigrated to countries across the sea.

(Cadwallader and some of his people went to Brittany). Then, Geoffrey continues:

> For eleven years Britain remained deserted by all its inhabitants, except for a few whom death had spared in certain parts of Wales. Even the Britons had come to hate their island; and it had no attraction for the Saxons, at this time, for they, too, kept dying there one after the other. However, once the deathly plague had ceased its ravages, those few Saxons who remained alive continued their age-old custom and sent a message to their fellow-countrymen in Germany to tell them that the island had been abandoned by its native population and would fall into

their hands without any difficulty at all, if only they would journey over to occupy it.

The account of plague in the Thorpe translation has no reference to any particular year for the simple reason that Geoffrey gives only three dates in his history: the death of Lucius in A.D. 156, the abdic on of Arthur in A.D. 542 and the death of Cadwallader in A.D. 689.

This epidemic has been commented upon by many writers and there is no evidence that it was bubonic plague. One feels, too, that there must have been some element of exaggeration in parts of this account. The death rate seems to have been excessive and it is difficult to imagine that Britain was so entirely deserted by its people even though some, like Cadwallader, did flee. Perhaps we should bear in mind the fact that there is doubt amongst scholars concerning the veracity, and even the authorship, of the work of Geoffrey of Monmouth and that it does not do to take all ancient works at their face value. Writing in 1190, less than forty years after Geoffrey's death, William of Newburgh said, 'It is quite clear that everything this man wrote about Arthur and his successors, or indeed about his predecessors from Vortigern onwards, was made up, partly by himself and partly by others, either from an inordinate love of lying, or for the sake of pleasing the Britons' (in Thorpe, 1966). As Thorpe says, 'In short, most of the material in the *History* really is fictional and someone did invent it'.

This epidemic was widespread over Europe and contemporary accounts spoke of its presence in Italy, Gaul and Spain. In about 691 Saint Adamnan wrote of:

> the plague, which in our times has twice devastated the greater part of the world. For not to mention the other and wider regions of Europe, namely Italy and the Roman city itself and the Cisalpine Provinces of the Gauls, also those of Spain, separated by the Pyrenean mountain range; the isles of the sea generally, namely, Ireland and Britain have been twice devastated by a dreadful pestilence, except two peoples, namely, the people of the Picts and that of the Scots of Britain, between whom the mountains of the Britannic Ridge [the Grampians] form a barrier.

It is interesting that this disease did not spread into the north whereas the fourteenth-century epidemic of bubonic plague was reported to have progressed into Scotland seemingly without hindrance, despite the severe effects of a harsh climate and a sparsely distributed human population upon the rat and the flea vectors.

It was recorded that the disease occurred especially in monasteries where the dirty conditions were said to favour its spread. Before towns grew, the monasteries were some of the larger communities of the population; the urban population being probably less than one-tenth of the total population. The chroniclers of the times were monks and it is to be expected that the outbreaks in the monasteries would receive careful attention. Another point which might be relevant is the age distribution of monks, whereby they would be either more or less prone to particular diseases. This question will be discussed when the disease of 1348–9 is examined. The movement of monks from one monastery to another was believed to help spread the infection although the accounts are not easy to evaluate. Clearly, however this disease killed many of the leading people of the time, most of whom were the senior members of monasteries.

To sum up this period and its epidemics is no easy matter but it seems clear that of the various diseases occurring in Britain between A.D. 545 and 667 none was bubonic plague. The medical evidence does not substantiate plague and Shrewsbury believes that most of these outbreaks were smallpox in 'virgin' societies. Macarthur (in Bonser, 1944) considered that Bede's plague, which began in A.D. 664, was bubonic in nature but there are few today who would agree with this. In assessing the true nature of *pestis flava* he considered it to be a severe form of relapsing fever with jaundice occurring as a complication and being common enough to dominate the general picture of the disease.

Between A.D. 667 and 1348 there were many epidemics but none of them can be identified as bubonic plague. Thus, of all the many outbreaks of disease recorded from the British Isles and elsewhere in the first thirteen and a half centuries, only one, the plague of Justinian, which did not reach Britain, can be confidently said to exhibit some of the characteristic symptoms of bubonic plague.

CHAPTER THREE

The Black Death – origins and spread to Europe

As there is no evidence for the presence of bubonic plague in the British Isles before 1348 it is improbable that there would have been a reservoir of dormant plague existing in any native or introduced rodent species. The disease had therefore to be transported from elsewhere, and as we now know from modern research, certain important factors enter into any consideration of the biological possibilities of such an event. There has been very little consideration of the biology of rats and fleas during the Black Death in particular and of bubonic plague in general in the British Isles and northern Europe.

Langer (1964) pointed out that today, when the threat of plague has been replaced by the threat of mass human extermination by modern warfare, there has been a renewal of interest in the history of the fourteenth-century epidemic. With the help of new perspectives, students are investigating its various effects: demographic, economic, psychological, moral and religious.

With the exception of demographic effects, these have all been studied regardless of what particular disease was involved because they are to a great extent independent of the biological processes of disease. As it has been long accepted that the epidemic of 1348–9 in Britain was bubonic plague, there was little reason for the historian or economist to question this: it was sufficient to know that the disease killed many people and that it occurred at a particular time. The results of the heavy mortality in terms of prices, labour shortage, moral attitudes and other effects all flowed from this calamity.

It is essential to examine the biological logistics of the Black Death to attempt to determine whether this particular epidemic could have been bubonic plague. In order to operate effectively that disease needs certain well-defined prerequisites involving rats, fleas, climate, human population density and even the structure of buildings. The carrying of plague over long distances by human activities is a feature about which we know something today but certain conditions are also necessary for this to take place. The accounts of the Black Death all describe how the disease came to Europe and the British Isles during a relatively short period of time; my purpose in this chapter is to examine the origin of the Black Death and the way it reached Europe, in the light of modern knowledge of plague biology.

Prior to the fourteenth century only the disease in the reign of Justinian, the symptoms of which were so carefully documented by Procopius, can be identified as bubonic plague although, as Shrewsbury has pointed out, other diseases were in evidence as well.

From the end of the sixth century until the middle of the fourteenth, nothing firmly identifiable as bubonic plague was heard of in the Mediterranean and southern Europe and speculation is fruitless in the absence of solid facts concerning rats and the various diseases then in evidence. However, the fact that plague died out in a relatively short space of time may encourage us to think that rats were either existing at low density, so low that they could not maintain enzootic plague, or were absent and that sylvatic plague, too, was presumably not present. The disease described by Procopius may have occurred in only a few areas in the eastern Mediterranean. The accounts of Gregory of Tours are less illuminating, and despite the strictures about accepting early accounts at face value, without adequate corroboration, Shrewsbury (1971) appears to accept that what Gregory described was in fact bubonic plague.

The brief appearance of plague in the Mediterranean in the sixth century was presumably a shift of the disease from one or other of the three old foci of plague. These were situated as follows:
(a) in the foothills of the Himalayas between India and China.
(b) in Central Africa in the region of the Great Lakes.
(c) scattered across the entire length of the Eurasian steppe from Manchuria to the Ukraine.
This last focus of endemic plague is the one from which the fourteenth-century pandemic could have developed. On geographical and trading grounds it looked likely and McNeill (1977) has argued that this reservoir is unlikely to be older than the fourteenth century A.D. He stresses the impact of the Mongol empire in the period A.D. 1200–1500 and points out that between A.D. 900 and 1200 communication patterns by land and sea altered. The Mongol empires founded by Genghis Khan embraced all China, nearly all Russia, central Asia, Iran and Iraq; overland caravan transport across Asia reached its climax during this time. Many people moved across Eurasia and McNeill claims that it was particularly important that a more northerly route came into use. Thus the Silk Road between China and Syria crossed the deserts of central Asia. The movements of traders between the Mongol headquarters at Karakorum and Kazan and Astrakhan on the Volga, Caffa in the Crimea, Khanbaliq in China and all points in between brought people into contact with the wild rodents of the steppes and McNeill speculates that the Mongol movements brought the bacteria of *Y. pestis* to the rodents of the Eurasian steppes.

The trade routes from the East were extensive and were first described in 1321 by Marinus Sanutus, a Venetian, in a work addressed to Pope John XXI (in Gasquet, 1908). The ancient centre of all trade with the far East was Bagdad, to which great city all the caravan routes led. There were two main lines of trade plus one other, perhaps longer, one. The first went from Bagdad over the plans of Mesopotamia and Syria to Lycia (the most southern part of Asiatic Turkey), where the goods were bought by Italian merchants. This was the shortest route for the produce of India and China to Europe but it was also the most perilous. The second line followed the Tigris to its sources in Armenia, then passed on, either to Trebizond and other ports of the Black Sea, or taking the road from the Caspian, upon the other side of the Caucasus, passed to Genoese and other flourishing settlements in the Crimea. The third route was the least dangerous. This went from India to ports in the Persian Gulf and then either by the Tigris route or to Aden. From there it went across the desert taking nine days to Chus (Kus, now Koos, near Thebes). Fifteen days on the Nile brought it to Cairo from where it went to Alexandria by canal.

Ziegler (1970) is of the opinion that the medieval pandemic began in central Asia. The Russian archaeologist Chwolson (1890) has shown an especially high death rate in 1338 and 1339 near Lake Issyk-Koul in the district of Semiriechinsk in central Asia; and Stewart (1928) in his account of the spread of Nestorian Christianity has drawn attention to two old cemeteries, fifty-five kilometres apart, which contained tombstones indicating they belonged to Nestorian Christians in Semiriechinsk. One of these graveyards contained 611 stones and for the years A.D. 1338–9 three inscriptions state that the persons buried had died of plague. He further pointed out that during those two years the number of inscriptions was exceptionally large. He also was of the opinion that plague originated in eastern Asia at about that time and that it spread rapidly to Asia Minor, North Africa and Europe and reached the Crimea in A.D. 1346.

Pollitzer (1954) has also referred to this large number of burials in the Nestorian graveyards and says quite categorically that it is therefore certain that plague was in evidence in central Asia a few years before the infection of the Crimean ports in 1346 and that from there it was carried by ship to Europe.

Many diseases were called plague and it seems that even if the term plague was used it has been taken by these authors as being, quite literally, bubonic plague. This would not satisfy the criteria of Shrewsbury. Another point of interest is the large number of inscriptions at the same time. These, presumably, had no such mention of plague otherwise note would have been made of this corroborative material. The abundance of inscriptions is not necessarily related to a plague epidemic although, for some reason or other, there appears to have been a high mortality. One wonders why only three stones gave the cause of death, although there were clearly many inscriptions.

Perhaps only the richer victims could afford elaborate inscriptions citing the cause of death or maybe in these three cases it was considered necessary because they died of something unusual.

Gasquet (1908) writes of a Prague chronicle which spoke of the epidemic in China, India and Persia and points out that although the plague epidemic was said to have originated in the East three or four years earlier, actual history can only trace its progress from the ports of the Black Sea, and possibly from those of the Mediterranean, to which traders along the main roads of commerce with Asiatic countries brought their merchandise for conveyance to the western world. The contemporary historian Matteo Villani reported that plague was conveyed to Europe by Italian traders who fled before it from ports on the eastern shores of the Black Sea. According to Gabriele de' Mussi, a notary of Piacenza, in the year 1346 in eastern parts an immense number of Tartars and Saracens fell victims to a mysterious and sudden death.

It is curious how many catastrophic happenings have been recorded from Asia in the thirteen years before plague was reported in Asia Minor in 1346. Drought, floods, earthquakes, famine, pestilence, swarms of locusts and so on, almost as though these were a necessary prelude to the crowning catastrophe of plague. Even if they actually occurred they were scattered over such a vast area in the greatest land mass in the world that it is unlikely that they would have had more than a local effect on either the fauna or disease patterns. On a smaller scale, the accounts of epidemics during Anglo-Saxon times in Britain frequently give details of a variety of extraordinary natural and supernatural events which preceded them. In the vast majority of the cases there is no causal relationship and it is quite likely that people thought back after events searching for portents, in accordance with the providential notion of disease and of history then prevalent.

Alarming accounts of some sort of epidemic in the East are given by Hecker (1859); 'India was depopulated, Tartary, Mesopotamia, Syria, Armenia were covered with dead bodies; the Kurds fled in vain to the mountains. In Caramania and Caesarea none were left alive.' There was almost certainly enormous exaggeration in some parts of this.

Hecker said that before the plague reached Europe it had killed daily, in Cairo, between 10,000 and 15,000 people, 'being as many as, in modern times, great plagues have carried off during their whole course'. More than 13,000,000 died in China. In Aleppo 500 died daily and within six weeks in Gaza 22,000 people and *most of the animals* were carried off (my italics). This is particularly noteworthy since bubonic plague has no record of killing animals other than rodents and men and some other agent may have been at work (see Chapter 11). If this was an accurate account it seems unlikely to have been bubonic plague.

It is very difficult to arrive at plague death figures from the more recent past, let alone the distant past, and taking Cairo as an example some very heavy mortality has been recorded. Sticker (1908) said that there were 860,000 deaths in 1574–6 and Alpinus (1591) reported 500,000 dead in the epidemic of 1581. As Petrie & Todd (1923) say, these estimates must be taken with much reserve. Russel (1791) was sceptical of the accuracy of the contemporary Egyptian figures and Aubert-Roche (1843) showed that the statistics compiled for the plague epidemics of 1834–5 in Alexandria were manipulated. One source of inaccuracy was the fact that plague occurred along with famine due to very low Nile floods; presumably, deaths were often wrongly assigned. Gaetani (1841) produced some of the most convincing records in his account of the Cairo epidemic of 1835, with a total of 33,751 deaths in six months.

What is also interesting is that, according to Hecker, plague was widespread in the land of the eastern Mediterranean and although the route of its introduction to Europe is said to be from the Crimea there may also have been parallel introductions from Syria since ships plied from there to the Italian and French ports. It would be a quicker journey by ship than from Odessa or other Black Sea ports and this factor may be important in the ability of plague to bridge the gap to the Italian mainland and thus become established in Europe.

Trade between Europe and the Crimea was well established and Vernadsky (1953) records that the Genoese seem to have penetrated into the Black Sea during the second half of the twelfth century. During the existence of the Latin Empire at Constantinople (1204–61), the Black Sea trade was almost entirely monopolised by the Venetians. One would imagine, therefore, that during this period there must have been, in addition to the passage of merchandise, a comparable transfer of disease organisms.

Gasquet (1908) says that from Caffa in the Crimea plague was probably carried to Constantinople where the Emperor John Cantacuzene described the epidemic which raged in northern Scythia in 1347. This pestilence reached almost all the sea-coasts, from which it was carried over to most of the Mediterranean world including Pontus, Thrace and Macedonia, Greece, Italy, the Islands, Egypt, Libya, Judea and Syria.

It is said that in the Crimea 85,000 died (Vernadsky, 1953). Ziegler records that, following a street fight, the local people turned on the Genoese who had a trading station at Tana and pursued the merchants to Caffa (now named Feodosia), the Genoese fortified base on the coast. The Tartars apparently laid siege to the town but plague broke out among their ranks and caused them to abandon the plan. Before leaving altogether they are said to have hurled some plague corpses into the city and although the Genoese disposed of them in the sea, they did not escape the plague which was soon active in the city. Realising that the depletion of numbers they were suffering would give them a poor chance against fresh Tartar attack they fled in their galleys towards the Mediterranean, taking plague with them.[3]

This episode, which was claimed to be the point of transfer of the Black Death to Europe, deserves a close analysis in terms of biological logistics. It is assumed that the beleaguered Genoese contracted plague from the Tartar corpses which were lobbed into them. If the bodies had died of bubonic plague then the only infective component would have been the rat flea or fleas which had previously infected the dead person. If such a flea had remained on a body until its death and stayed on it afterwards then it might have left the corpse and bitten one of the city people; but it is more likely that it would have left the body much earlier, as it cooled, before it was thrown into the city, and infected one of the Tartars. Medical and biological evidence is against infection in the manner suggested. A corpse resulting from bubonic plague is itself no hazard to people around it because the post mortem processes of autolysis of tissues are sufficient quickly to render the bacteria harmless.

The human flea, *Pulex irritans*, may have been on the body before death, and whilst it is occasionally possible for this flea to transmit plague, it has been shown that in normal bubonic infections there are insufficient bacilli in the blood of the patient to render a flea infective, although this may be possible in the rather less frequent cases of septicaemic plague. The final variation is that the Tartars may have been in the throes of a pneumonic plague outbreak. Even so, bacilli in the lungs would be inactivated soon after death and from the evidence presented later (p. 162) it is hard to see how infections resulting from corpses would take place. It seems more likely that if plague was present inside Caffa it arose from sources such as rats within the city walls. Since, as Ziegler points out, plague was probably in the general area then the commensal rodents would be a more realistic focus of infection.

Whatever the cause of the infection within the city, it would be natural for the defenders to attribute it to the corpses thrown in, in view of the state of contemporary medical knowledge, and for the same reasons a legitimate tactic for the besieging forces to adopt. Without better information, which is unlikely to be forthcoming, we shall never know the extent of plague in the beseiged town. The story has it that the survivors took to the sea and headed for home, presumably taking plague along with them by some means or other, since these same galleys are said to have brought it to the seaports of southern Europe. De Smet recounted that in January 1348, three galleys put in at Genoa. These had been driven by a strong wind from the East, were seriously infected and were laden with a variety of spices and other valuable goods. 'When the inhabitants of Genoa learnt this, and saw how suddenly and irremediably they infected other people, they were driven forth from that port by burning arrows and divers engines of war; for no man dared touch them; nor was any man able to trade with them, for if he did he would be sure to die forthwith. Thus, they were scattered from port to port.'

Commenting on this, Ziegler points out that by the time the Genoese authorities reacted to this threat it was already too late and the infection was established on shore. By the spring of 1348 the Black Death was firmly entrenched both in Sicily and on the mainland, having arrived in Sicily early in October 1347. Michael of Piazza, writing ten years later, said that twelve

Genoese galleys brought plague to Messina. No one knows where they came from but Ziegler comments that if, as seems likely, they came from the Crimea then they must have left that region several months before those ships which carried plague from Caffa to Genoa and Venice. His added comment is interesting: 'No one can now know whether the disease was borne by rats and fleas or was already rampant among members of the crew; the chroniclers description of "sickness clinging to their very bones" suggests the latter. Within a few days the plague had taken a firm grasp on the city.' At this point the people of Messina drove the ships from the port and 'with their going, the Black Death was scattered around the Mediterranean'. Apparently, hundreds of people were dying each day in Messina, 'the slightest contact with the sick seeming a guarantee of rapid infection'. The population of the city fled and spread plague through the countryside. Thus runs the account of the origin of plague's introduction into Europe. I shall return later to look at the events on land, but before doing so the means by which plague came by sea from the Crimea must be examined. If this was the route then we must be sure that it was biologically possible.

One of the important points to consider in this account of plague transfer is the type of ship plying between Genoa and the Crimean ports. It is necessary to know the size of the vessel, how many crew and passengers, the quantity of cargo and the time taken to make the journey. All these factors are of importance in determining whether plague could survive in rats or people and still begin a severe epidemic immediately on reaching its destination.

During the twelfth and thirteenth centuries commerce grew in the Mediterranean. Larger, costlier and more efficient ships were developed to cope with the increasing numbers of merchants, extra cargo, pilgrims and the Crusaders with their horses and weapons. There were three main types of vessel: the sailing ship; the galley driven by oars with up to three masts, but usually one or two and as many sails for assistance in lights winds; and the *tarida*, which was slower and heavier than a galley. This latter had oars and two masts with a full set of sails on each mast. Byrne (1930) in his monograph on Genoese shipping says that, contrary to impressions given by many writers, most overseas commerce was carried in sailing ships until near the end of the thirteenth century. For the short haul of merchandise in gross between Genoa and trade centres near Genoa, galleys which were decked over were used. They carried cloth in bulk from southern French ports and eastern wares to Sicily and Barcelona. By the end of the century when the movements of Crusaders and pilgrims to the East slowed down, galleys became used more generally for trade with the Levant and Flanders. Their advantages were that they were faster, cheaper and easier to defend. The *tarida*, a slower vessel than the other two, carried the horses and food of the Crusaders and shipped grain, meat, cheese and such heavy goods.

In the thirteenth century ships were quite large. Some Venetian ships were 110 feet overall, with a maximum beam of 41 feet, and the largest Genoese ship was just over 83 feet. One of the largest vessels built in Genoa for St Louis carried four ship's boats (three was usual) of which the greatest was equipped with 52 oars. Large vessels could carry 100 horses along with Crusaders and servants, and this type of vessel, when engaged in ordinary voyages, could accommodate over a thousand passengers. Byrne cites evidence from a Genoese document of 1248 in which the owner of a ship states that he was sold 1100 places on a ship bound for Syria. This particular vessel was not extraordinarily large as she carried 75 sailors plus officers and servants, whereas some ships needed 100. When a thousand or more passengers were carried most would be pilgrims and it was not considered necessary to give them much space.

There is little information on cargo capacity but from the scanty data available Byrne considered that 600 tons, dead cargo weight, was probably near the maximum for Genoese ships at this time. He does point out that on a longer, more hazardous voyage such as to the Levant, the cargo might have been less. It is interesting that Spanish, English and Dutch merchant vessels engaged in transoceanic trade in the sixteenth century carried between 600 and 800 tons.

This information on Genoese vessels holds good for the late thirteenth century and there is no evidence that any marked changes had taken place in the next 100 years. Thus, ships were large and, as the decked over galleys had extended their range by the end of the thirteenth century, the reports of galleys plying between Genoa and the Crimea are doubtless accurate.

On ships the size of these it would be possible to carry a considerable number of rats within the cargo and within the ships' fabric. Even without large numbers of pilgrims the number of crew and merchants would ensure that large quantities of food would have to be carried for the journey. We have very little knowledge of the absolute size of rat populations on board ships today, even after fumigation, because so few bodies are recovered. During the early years of this century when plague was active in Egypt the investigators searched feluccas, the Nile sailing boats, to determine whether they harboured rodents and fleas and might thus aid the spread of plague (Petrie & Todd, 1923). Feluccas are built with an inner and outer planking bolted to the cross-ribs and this provides a hollow space in which rats can find shelter. Between January and December 1912, 278 feluccas moored at El Hamra were each trapped twice on average. 216 of them yielded rodents, a total of 683 animals from four species:

Rattus norvegicus	495
Rattus rattus	127
Acomys cahirinus	57
Arvicanthis niloticus	4

Equally important is the number of fleas on the rodents, since without them plague will not be transmitted. Flea counts on the trapped rodents showed the following:

	Average no. fleas/rodent
A. niloticus	0
R. norvegicus	29.4
R. rattus	14.0

Each felucca carried two or three crew and there were seven passengers per 100 boats. The number of rats caught bore no relation to the nature of the cargo, whether edible or non-edible, carried at the time of trapping. This observation indicated that the infesting rodents were not merely travellers but were actual colonists in the boats.

The galleys could therefore presumably support many rats. A large population would be necessary for there to be a sufficient number of plague-infected rats with fleas to survive, at worst, an epizootic on the voyage and for enough of the vectors to arrive in Genoa or Messina and escape ashore to infect the local rats, a proceeding which is neither so swift nor so easy as many writers have believed.

The maintenance of plague on board ship during a long journey, with enough non-immune rats and their fleas alive to come ashore and yet at the same time with enough crew also remaining alive is a difficult biological balancing act. All the accounts of the arrival of plague on the European mainland or Sicily speak of the disease spreading fast almost as soon as docking took place. If this was so then plague had taken place late in the voyage. However, the Genoese left Caffa because plague was active there at the time and they presumably took plague-infected rats on board. This should have ensured that plague occurred early in the voyage as the rats died and their fleas took to men. If plague occurred early then many crew must have died, the remainder either escaping or becoming immune, the shipboard rats also dying or surviving and becoming immune. It is important to remember that bubonic plague does not occur in man unless there is an epizootic amongst rats, nor does pneumonic plague usually occur from rats without there first being bubonic cases.

The distance from Caffa to Messina is about 1600 miles by the shortest route and to Genoa 2200 miles. Most sea travel took place between May and October, partly on account of the winter storms and also because the overcast skies of winter made navigation difficult since, until the compass was invented, mariners plotted courses by landmarks or the sun by day, and the stars at night. Sailing in winter was mainly dictated by emergencies and the flight from Caffa which reached Genoa in January would have been in this category.

The time a voyage took depended on the winds and as most sea crossings took place in the summer months the summer trade winds would determine the speed. These blow steadily from the north and would aid such journeys as those from Rome to Alexandria (1400 miles) which in the summer might take between 10 and 21 days, but the return journey could take two months or more. Pliny records journeys of six and seven days from the Straits of Messina to Alexandria and tells how the praetorian senator Valerius Matianus made Alexandria from Pozzuoli in nine days with a very gentle breeze. It is difficult to calculate how long the galleys would have taken from Caffa to Genoa. In Greek and Roman times journeys across the Mediterranean in a fairly straight line, and presumably with favourable winds, varied from 50 to 140 miles per day, e.g. Rome to Alexandria op. cit. The return journey against head winds would only average around 25 miles per day.

The voyage from the Crimea to Italy is far from being an easy one. The navigation of the Aegean Sea is difficult and the direction of the journey changes from south-west to west with finally a long haul northwards to Genoa. A favourable wind over some part of the journey is likely to be unfavourable over the rest of it, slowing down the average daily progress. Allowing for these difficulties and taking a daily mileage somewhere between the two extremes mentioned it seems unlikely that any voyage could have been completed in less than four or five weeks. At worst, based on 25 miles per day, it could have been as long as 85 days, almost three months.

With journeys of this duration there is little doubt that in the confined quarters of a ship, plague, if it became epizootic amongst rats, would be distributed to the sailors in a fairly short time as hungry 'blocked' fleas sought new hosts, the surviving rats and men being immune and offering no danger to shore-based populations on landing. Certainly, some of the accounts of the arrival of plague in Europe do not stand up to careful analysis. For example, Creighton (1894) says that the Italian traders escaped the plague, yet 'the infection appeared in Genoa in its most deadly form a day or two after the arrival of the ship, although none of those on board were suffering from the plague'. He is quite adamant on this point and elsewhere repeats it emphatically, saying, 'for we know that there were no cases of plague on board ships, although the very atmosphere or smell of the new arrival seemed sufficient to taint the whole air of Genoa and *to carry death to every part of the city within a couple of days*'.

This, if the disease was bubonic plague, is highly improbable. In the first place it is unlikely that there were no shipboard infections if plague was so available on docking. Secondly, even if infected rats or crew had come ashore, the shore epidemic would not have started so soon, let alone spread with such rapidity. People suffering from bubonic plague on landing would present little health hazard and would certainly not create an epidemic of the proportions claimed. Non-immune, infected rats too would be of little danger until they had begun an epizootic which in due course would be seen in the spread to the human population. As I shall show in later chapters the spread of plague in modern times has been a relatively slow business initially and we have no good reason to suppose that it was any different in the fourteenth century. Whatever differences there may have been in the virulence of the bacillus are to a great extent irrelevant because its spread then, as today, would still be dependent upon the presence of adequate numbers of rats and fleas. Indeed, where modern writers have suggested that the plague was of an especially virulent nature in the Black Death they have overlooked the fact that excessive virulence, while leading to high and quick mortality, may also lead to a rapid end to the epidemic because it will kill off all the maintenance hosts – the rats – in whom continuous propagation is essential for plague to continue.

Neither the contemporary accounts of how the plague reached southern Europe nor some of the modern versions of the situation are, therefore, very convincing when we consider the facts in the light of the behaviour of known plague. It is certain that a disease was introduced – it is by no means clear what that disease was.

CHAPTER FOUR

The disease in Europe

The disease, which is said to have been plague and was carried from the Crimea, seems to have enjoyed a curious and unique duality in its powers. It could travel over two thousand miles on a small ship where rats, fleas and men would have been in close proximity and according to one report (Creighton, 1894) no one on board was infected, yet the moment it reached harbour it swept through a city in two days. When the galleys were sent back to sea their crews were able to sail to Marseilles and on to Spain 'leaving a trail of infection along the coast of Languedoc'. Furthermore, this highly selective organism which destroyed land dwellers but spared mariners was carrying out this destruction of life in the winter months. The Genoese would, at the earliest, have left Caffa during October and at the latest by December. Flea breeding must have been very low at that time both on ship and ashore and the speed of spread in Genoa was so fast that it is difficult to imagine even influenza going through a city in that way. Pneumonic plague is often assumed to have been rife in the medieval pandemic yet there is little unequivocal evidence of its presence and modern data on its spreading capacity do not support the view. In any case, in murine plague pneumonic arises from primary cases of bubonic plague, to initiate which there must be rats and fleas.

Even in the absence of rats, when blocked fleas have travelled in merchandise the spread of plague is not sudden and follows a time scale such as that briefly outlined in Chapter 1, p. 21, and described in detail from modern epidemics in Chapter 8. The Genoa illness, if accurately reported, resembled neither plague nor any other disease that we know today if it spread at that speed. In those days and even in more recent times before the advent of air travel, many diseases were introduced to ports and from there spread inland along whatever communications existed. In this century plague itself has been introduced to many countries in this way, infected rats from ships' cargoes infesting the dockyards and spreading infection to people, local rats and, eventually, the endemic non-murine rodents.

Ziegler (1970) says that three great centres for the propagation of plague in southern Europe were Sicily, Genoa and Venice, plague arriving more or less simultaneously in Genoa and Venice in January, 1348. Pisa, which was attacked a few weeks later, was the main point of entry to central and northern Italy, plague moving rapidly inland to Rome and Tuscany. In relation to the spread of plague he goes on, 'the Black Death, indeed, is peculiar among plagues in that the *particularly high incidence of its pneumonic variant* meant that it struck inland with unusual vigour'. We have little real evidence of when or where it was in the pneumonic form.

The first pandemic did not spread across Europe because, presumably, there was a lack of *Rattus rattus*. It is generally assumed, though, that by 1347 this species was widespread in Europe and hence plague was able to spread freely to all parts. Ziegler says that there is no doubt that the rapid spread of bubonic plague was greatly helped by the presence of infected rats and that there was no shortage of them, maintaining that by the middle of the fourteenth century they were abundant in Europe, having probably arrived in the boats of the returning Crusaders.

The disease reached Marseilles in February 1348, and it has been said that as many as 56,000 died. Whatever the cause, mortality was greater than in the inland regions. It must be mainly speculation that the two forms, bubonic and pneumonic, were active at the same time. Ziegler (1970) gives some account of the death rates due to plague in parts of rural France. In Givry, a Burgundian village of between 1,200 and 1,500 people near Chalon-sur-Saône, 30 deaths per year were recorded in the years preceding the Black Death but between 5 August and 19 November, 1348, as many as 615 died. In 1347 in Saint-Pierre-du-Soucy in Savoy the 108 households were reduced to 68 by the end of 1348 and to 55 in 1349. In seven neighbouring parishes the number of households fell from 303 to 142 and Ziegler comments that in such rural areas close on 50 per cent of the population must have died.

According to Hankin (1905) the intensity of a plague outbreak in India was in inverse proportion to the size of the community, the maximum mortality being in villages rather than towns. He gives some data in support of this during the plague outbreaks occurring between 1897 and 1898:

Place	Population	Death rate per 1000
Bombay	806,144	20.1
Poona	161,696	31.2
Karachi	97,009	24.1
Sholapur	61,564	35.0
Kale	4,431	104.9
Supne	2,068	102.5
Ibrampur	1,692	360.5

He further maintained that though plague spread with facility from a town or village to a neighbouring village it did not often appear to be carried to great distances in epidemic form. Although this might well have been true for India the constraints of climate and other factors might have resulted in a different situation in northern Europe.

From Marseilles the disease went west to Montpellier and Narbonne, reaching Carcassone between February and May, progressing to Toulouse and Montauban and arriving in Bordeaux in August. According to Biraben (1975) and Langer (1964) (Fig. 4) it had reached Bordeaux before June 1348.

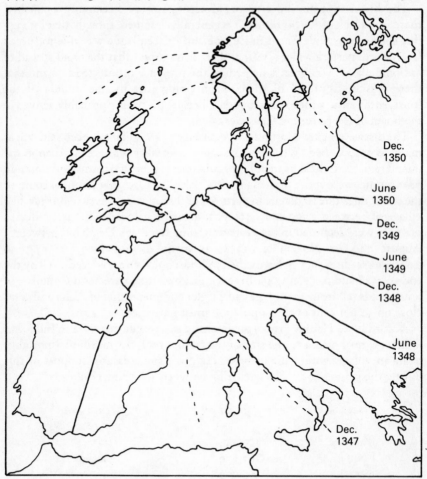

Fig. 4 The spread of the Black Death across Europe in the fourteenth century (after Langer, 1964)

In a northerly direction the infection appeared in Avignon in March, April and May, Lyons in early summer, Paris in June and Burgundy in July and August. From Paris, according to Gasquet (1908), the pestilence divided, one stream going through Normandy towards the coast which it probably reached in the area round Calais about July or August 1348 (he says about 25

July, the Feast of St James) whilst the other stream, which was said to be checked by autumn and winter, made its way less rapidly towards Belgium and Holland.

When we look at the later spread of known plague in more recent times this is a remarkably swift passage. If it is assumed that rat populations were contiguous throughout the region – and they would need to have been – then the rate of spread across France is as follows:

Marseilles to Carcassone – five miles per day
Carcassone to Bordeaux – one and a half or three miles per day depending which
version one follows
Marseilles to Avignon – one and a half miles per day
Avignon to Lyons – two miles per day
Marseilles to Paris – two and a half miles per day

In Figure 4 it can be seen that the advance of the disease, if it progressed as a steadily spreading infection, was rapid in the early stages from early 1348 (or December 1347) up to June 1348, covering much of France and Spain, crossing the Alps and covering Italy, and a large slice of the Balkans.

Gasquet (1908) says that plague spread north along the mountain passes, by way of the Brenner Pass to Bavaria, along the St Gothard Pass and the Rhine Valley and up the Rhône Valley to Switzerland from France. By June it was in Bavaria and by December 1348, had reached northern Germany. Thereafter, the advance of the disease front was generally substantially less for each six monthly period, with the exception of Spain and perhaps the British Isles between June and December, 1349.

On the continent of Europe certain places, either partially or totally, escaped the epidemic. Of the towns, Milan, Liége and Nuremberg were free of the disease. A small area towards the north-west end of the Pyrenees is said to have avoided plague although it seems very strange that the disease was present over the rest of the mountain range. Another small area east of Calais also escaped and, even more interestingly, a very large area north of Vienna. This region was roughly the same size as England and if it was completely plague-free it is curious because it is in an area where the climate is continental and where one would expect the summer temperatures to be high enough to encourage flea breeding. On the other hand, the disease spread freely across the Alps and Pyrenees and across Norway, Sweden and far east into the Baltic, all areas which provide especially poor conditions for *Rattus rattus*. As I shall show later, even in the climatically warmer parts of the region the conditions were poor for an animal which is so dependent upon warmth.

The disease reached England at a point thought to be Melcombe Regis, now part of Weymouth, although some early chroniclers believed that it first appeared in Bristol and Southampton. The date of arrival is even more in dispute, although there is fairly general agreement that it was during late June or July. According to one account it reached Dorset a little before the Feast of

St John the Baptist, i.e. before 24 June 1348 and according to another the plague began about St Peter's Day, 29 June. Other dates given are 7 and 25 July and Robert of Avesbury gives the beginning of August. One source claims it arrived in the autumn of 1348.

There can only be speculation about where it came from. The south coast of England had shipping arriving from Calais, northern French ports and the Channel Islands as well as from the Baltic, the Atlantic seaboard of France and from the Mediterranean. As the disease was probably present in all but the Baltic, it might have come from any of these sites. However, in 1348 Calais was in the possession of the English so that ships no doubt crossed regularly to English ports. At that time Melcombe Regis was a busy port, evidenced by the fact that in 1347–8 it furnished Edward III with 20 ships and 264 marines for his siege of Calais.

After the introduction into England through Weymouth it becomes difficult to chart the actual routes by which the disease progressed across Britain. It is said that during the initial stages of its invasion it was restricted to the south-western ports, from each of which it would radiate for some distance inland, and was carried along the coast by boats (Shrewsbury, 1971). Bristol was the first town of importance to be infected. According to Boucher (1938) plague reached Melcombe on 1 August and Bristol on 15 August. If it proceeded overland from one to the other it would have covered close on five miles per day. Shrewsbury, using the dates of introduction given by Robert of Avesbury and Galfridi le Baker (i.e. the beginning of August) says that it took 47 days to reach Bristol, a rate of passage of one and a half miles per day, closely corresponding, he says, to the time taken to spread from Marseilles to Paris and Bristol to London. Shrewsbury says that there is general agreement among contemporary chroniclers that plague appeared in Marseilles about Christmas 1347 and that Klebs asserts that it broke out in Paris soon after October 1348 and not in midsummer as is still frequently stated in the literature. If these dates are correct he comments that plague took more than ten months to travel overland the 400-odd miles between these two cities.

A rate of one and a half miles per day is too slow, according to Shrewsbury, to support the supposition that plague was carried on land in goods which contained 'blocked' fleas because even the clumsiest of fourteenth-century goods wagons would cover 10–12 miles a day in summer. His estimate that it would on that basis reach Bristol within ten days of leaving Melcombe Regis is at variance with the mileage of 69 he gives and also with the estimate of wagons taking 14 days to travel from Bristol to London. Based on 10 to 12 miles a day more realistic times would be five and a half days and nine or ten days for Melcombe to Bristol and Bristol to London respectively.

The alternative suggestion is that plague must have spread from Melcombe to Bristol either as a creeping epizootic by rat to rat contacts or, more likely, by coastal shipping. As Shrewsbury points out, it would be more profitable to take bulky cargoes by sea than to unload them at Melcombe Regis and haul them overland. His suggestion that the spread of disease might have been by a creeping epizootic is interesting because of its implication that *Rattus rattus* was widespread across the countryside. Even if rats had been as numerous as this, recent experience has shown that plague would not have spread as quickly as it did, not even at one and a half miles per day.

In addition to manorial records which give information about the mortality of the general population, much of the information on the presence and severity of the epidemic in Britain has been gleaned from Church records which show the Institutions to benefices made empty because the incumbent had vacated the living, the assumption often being that he had died of plague. The proportion of priests replaced to those remaining unaffected has been extrapolated to the population as a whole and many mortality estimates are based on this information. It is by no means certain, however, that priests ran the same risk as parishioners. If they were zealous they may have been in greater danger from a highly infectious disease but on the other hand those who hesitated to visit the sick when the pestilence was raging might have had a lower incidence of sickness. Furthermore, from the evidence gleaned during the modern pandemic, it is now clear that attendance upon those sick with bubonic plague carries little risk of infection (p. 162). Thus an accurate identification of the disease responsible for the Black Death might aid us in assessing the relative risks of priest and parishioner.

It is generally accepted that the vacation of a benefice automatically implies the death of the incumbent and some writers have assumed that all vacations during 1348–9 were due to death from plague. However, Thompson (1947) has pointed out that during the fourteenth century a custom of exchanging ecclesiastical benefices had reached serious proportions and that by the end of the century it had developed into an abuse. There existed brokers who arranged these exchanges and the existence of these people caused Archbishop Courtenay to issue a strongly worded mandate against what he called 'chop-churches' in 1392.

Thompson gives some examples of such exchanges: when Thomas Hexham died in the deanery of Chester-le-Street in 1408, John Thoralby had collation on 6 April but on 12 April exchanged for the rectory of Lockington, in the East Riding of Yorkshire, with John Dalton, an official of Bishop Langley. On 15 April Dalton resigned. He had accepted the vacant deanery of Lanchester and was succeeded at Chester-le-Street the next day by Walter Bosum. Two weeks later, on 1 May Bosum exchanged the deanery for the vicarage of St Oswald's, Durham, with Robert Assheburn who held the post until his death in 1412–13. Another example was of a resignation by Thomas del Hay in 1411 and collation by Robert del Hay on 27 December. On 22 January 1412 Robert exchanged this situation with Thomas for one in Howden but Thomas resigned it on 13 March and next day Robert again had collation. If these bewildering series of exchanges have been recorded in diocesan records one cannot help wondering whether figures for Institutions may not in some cases have been inflated since at face value they could imply a disease of alarming severity. Some registers, however, enable us to separate deaths of incumbents from vacancies due to other causes.

Be this as it may, the records show times when replacements greatly exceeded the normal rate and with caution these records may be used in studying the period when the disease was active. According to Fletcher (1922), who amended the figures given by Cardinal Gasquet (1908), the plague caused the following Institutions in the period October 1348 until August 1349 in Dorset:

> October (4): November (17): December (28) – the peak: January (21): February (12): March (12): April (6).

This makes a total of 100. The previous average had been one a month. The disease carried on until August and during these four months the Institutions were:

> May (9): June (3): July (11): August (5).

If all these deaths were due to plague there is a clear peak in the depths of winter, December and January, and summer figures are lower than winter ones. Fletcher states that the parts of the county most affected were the districts within a short distance of the coast and the villages through which the River Winterbourne passes before emptying itself into the Stour. He goes on to point out that from 24 June until Christmas it rained either by day or by night almost without exception and concluded that the abnormally wet season would aid the development of the sickness. In fact this would have made it cooler than in a dry season and conditions for flea breeding would be adverse, if it was bubonic plague. Both *Rattus rattus* and *Xenopsylla cheopis* dislike damp, cold weather. Fletcher, quoting from Gasquet (1908) and Hecker (1859), says that the plague which was some form of the ordinary Eastern or bubonic plague, showed itself in swellings and carbuncles under the arm and in the groin – sometimes as large as a hen's egg but sometimes smaller and distributed over the body. In addition he draws attention to special symptoms, from one or more of which the patient suffered and these seemed to differentiate it from the common type. These were: gangrenous inflammation of the throat and lungs, violent pains in the chest, the vomiting and spitting of blood and a pestilential odour coming from the bodies and breath of the sick. He goes on to say that though many recovered from the carbuncles and glandular swellings, none did from the blood spitting.

This account must be treated with extreme caution because it is a perfect example of how, on so many occasions, modern chroniclers of the Black Death have presented features for which there is little or no evidence. Fletcher's account is taken largely from Hecker (1859), but he has omitted to point out that these special symptoms were those documented by the Emperor John Cantakusene of Constantinople who had pointed out that these additional symptoms had not been connected with the oriental plague before. As I shall detail later (Chapter 11), Hecker draws attention to the disease in the West where a quite different set of symptoms was in evidence. Thus, Fletcher has not given the symptoms of the disease in Dorset but has accepted that bubonic plague was present and then fitted plague details from Hecker's general account to substantiate the disease. The disease in Dorset lasted for nearly 12 months, increasing in intensity until the end of the spring of 1349, then slowly decreasing.

According to Rees (1920) the Black Death spread to Wales by way of the Severn valley into the border counties and into the lordships of south-eastern March. Previous to the winter or spring of 1348–9 the records showed no sign of anything out of the ordinary but by March the epidemic was raging in the eastern and western portion of the lordship of Bergavenny and by the middle of April 'almost wholesale destruction had been wrought among the inhabitants', only one-third of the original rents being obtained in most hamlets. It should perhaps be pointed out here that non-payment of rents was not due solely to deaths for there are many examples after 1348 of refusal to pay rents because they were too high now that land was no longer scarce. The attempt on the part of landowners to continue on a pre-plague basis led to much bad feeling which finally culminated in the Peasants' Revolt.

Many parts of Wales were affected and although there was no direct evidence of pestilence in Brecon and Huntington, receipts showed greater fluctuation than in ordinary years. Rees, however, gives no data on comparisons of the years of pestilence with ordinary years. In north-east Wales, Rhuddlan, Holywell and Flint were all affected, the lordship of Denbigh being especially badly hit. Many of the lead miners of Holywell died and those surviving refused to carry on working there.

The Court Rolls for Ruthin are good and show that from January to May, 1349 inclusive, there were the usual court proceedings. Then suddenly in the second week in June there were seven deaths within the jurisdiction of the Court of Abergwiller and during the next two weeks all parts of the lordship were seriously attacked. During that brief period, 77 people of the town of Ruthin died. In the neighbourhood of Llangollen, ten died, Llanerch had 13 deaths, Dogfelen 25 and Abergwiller 14, figures which more than doubled in the next few weeks.

By the last week of July or early August the epidemic had abated, only to break out with renewed violence during the remainder of August when the death rate reached its highest. It then fell rapidly, although a few deaths were attributed to plague throughout the following winter. About the end of March, Carmarthen had early victims (the Carmarthen district suffered severely at this first visitation) and during the summer the pestilence made serious ravages throughout the administrative districts of Ystrad Towy and Cardigan.

There was a heavier toll of victims in the Principality of North Wales than in the South, a curious feature for a disease dependent upon the distribution of the Black rat. Caernarvon suffered serious losses, Anglesey probably likewise, and almost all the villeins of Deganwy died but by the end of 1349 the epidemic had generally subsided.

From Bristol the pestilence probably went eastwards into Oxfordshire, Berkshire and Buckinghamshire. Details of actual routes of spread are too imprecise from now on although we can see a general forward movement of the disease eastwards and northwards across the British Isles. Whatever it was it moved very swiftly. For example, in the Hundred of Farnham in Surrey, 20 miles south-south-east of Reading, it was estimated that from the number of holdings becoming vacant each month the disease probably arrived in the autumn of 1348. In this Hundred there were several holdings vacant in December, then there was a low period but the months of June and September, 1349, had several vacancies. The Institutions in Surrey, however, did not reach a maximum until May, 1349 as the following shows: January (5); February (8); March (12); April (12); May (23); June (6); July (7); August (2); September (5). In Oxfordshire the worst period was March, April and May 1349.

The disease probably progressed from Southampton and the West Country across Hampshire, Wiltshire and Surrey towards London. The epidemic is said to have reached Bodmin in the west just before Christmas 1348 and London at Michaelmas or All Saints (1 November). If it reached London from Bristol via Oxford, as is thought to be the case, and it did not make its first appearance in Bristol until mid August, then it must have made the journey of 100 miles in under two months, a rate of just under two miles a day. Although there were cases as early as November 1348 in London, the main epidemic began early in 1349, reaching a peak after Candlemas (2 February) 1349 and ending by Pentecost (Whitsuntide Sunday) of that year. Ziegler comments that perhaps between 20,000 and 30,000 died in this epidemic. This is probably too high an estimate since the population in 1348 before plague was not far from 60,000 according to Russell (1948). Up to 1349 the epidemic progressed from the south-west by two main lines to London and the Thames Valley, although after March 1349 the infection did not advance regularly but sprang up simultaneously in many places. Throughout East Anglia – including Cambridgeshire, Norfolk, Suffolk and north Essex – the epidemic arrived in May 1349 and also reached York on 21 May, having taken about ten months to travel from south Dorset. At a very rough calculation the overall rate of spread was something in the region of 25 miles per month, a little over one mile a day.

Estimates of mortality in the several dioceses of England have been given considerable attention. It is probably unfortunate that the diocese has been treated as a unit because its size is often very considerable and it may cover many different types of land usage, as well as moorland and town. However, without the church-based records our knowledge of the epidemic would be even more scanty (although as indicated above estimations of death rates based solely on Institutions to new benefices should be treated with caution).

Diseases vary to some extent in the mortality rates of specific age classes and if this information is available and is accurate it can be of some assistance in helping to narrow the field in the identification of past epidemics. Russell (1948) took information from the Inquisitions *Post Mortem*, an unfortunately small sample, for four epidemic periods in the fourteenth century, beginning with 1348–50 and these data are presented in Table 1. In 1348–50 the one to five age group has a high death rate whilst the six to ten class has the lowest. Between age 11 and 30 the death rate is roughly similar and is fairly high in the 31 to 65 classes. With the exception of the youngest group, one to five year olds, the mortality broadly increases with age.

TABLE 1

Age specific mortality of the four epidemics of the fourteenth century

(the figures represent the percentage dying of plague at each age group). Data from Russell (1948) taken from the Inquisitions *Post Mortem*.

Age	1348–1350	1360–1	1369	1375
1–5	33	20	–	0
6–10	7	10	20	0
11–15	15	11	15	5
16–20	20	17	14	11
21–25	20	22	3	16
26–30	19	22	14	16
31–35	28	13	2	6
36–40	33	21	15	13
41–45	21	22	21	7
46–50	29	33	12	3
51–55	34	18	14	12
56–60	46	41	5	15
61–65	39 (over 60)	38	31	27
Above 65	–	33	15	33

The data of the Plague Research Commission (1907) of known bubonic plague deaths in Bombay city in the early part of the twentieth century show a very different age mortality, as can be seen below (the death rates are expressed as the incidence per 1000 for each age period with percentages in parentheses alongside):

Age	Incidence/1000	Percentage
Above 60	3.8	(0.38)
41–60	7.2	(0.72)
21–40	10.6	(1.06)
11–20	18.7	(1.87)
6–10	12.6	(1.26)
0–5	3.4	(0.34)

It is clear without any elaboration that there is considerable difference between these two disease mortality patterns.

Russell's data for the other three plagues of the fourteenth century, namely 1360–1, 1369 and 1375 (Table 1) indicate that the higher mortality rates are usually found in the upper age groups although in two cases (1360–1 and 1369) there is a fall in the over 65 age group. In 1360–1 the lowest mortality occurs in age groups six to 20 but is, however, high in the under fives. In 1369 the 11–15 group does not have a death rate that is lower than other groups. In fact it is very similar to six or seven other age groups and the six to ten year olds have a fairly high mortality. In 1375, not only do all the under 15s have a low mortality but also the age groups 31–35, 41–45 and 46–50.

Philip and Hirst (1917) studied an outbreak of plague in Colombo and reported that the largest number of cases occurred in people between the ages of ten and 25, with the very young and the elderly being comparatively slightly affected. Pointing out that a similar incidence was seen in India they surmised that it was probable that those at the extremes of life were less susceptible than full-blooded young adults. In the light of the Bombay and Ceylon figures, the death rates of the age classes from the fourteenth-century epidemics might indicate that diseases other than bubonic plague and with different mortality patterns were also present.

Russell (1968) makes some curious deductions stemming from the death rate when, for example, he says that in the plague in England in 1348–50 the death rate among both clergy and older men was high, with scholars also suffering heavily. He attributes this high death rate in smaller households to the fact that there would be more flea contacts than in larger households. The smallest households were those of the peasants (see Chapter 6), whilst one would expect scholars and clergy to either live in larger houses or in monasteries. In any event we have no means of knowing who was likely to experience more flea contacts. Russell's conclusions, based on his belief that the plague mortality rate among beneficed clergy was higher because they were older and therefore subject to a higher mortality, may need some revision in the light of modern knowledge that older people were *less* likely to suffer from plague.

Shrewsbury adds to the clamour for impossible evidence from the past when he says that no historian has attempted to show how the homes of beneficed clergy and the cottages of common folk compared with respect to their rat infestations in the fourteenth century. He maintains that until evidence is presented to show that the dwellings of the clergy were more rat-infested than those of their parishioners, there can be no justification for assuming that as a class they suffered any more severely from bubonic plague than the members of equivalent classes in that society. There is not even a remote chance of ever knowing this and it is most unlikely that we could learn much about it in objective terms for such dwellings 100 years ago, let alone well over 600 years.

Before the epidemic (see Russell, 1948: Fig. 17, Chapter 10), the monthly mortality records showed two peaks: one in January–February and the other in October–November with a minimum in June and July. According to Shrewsbury the winter peak was due to deaths from smallpox, typhus fever and infections of the respiratory tract and the autumn one to deaths from diphtheria, measles, St Anthony's Fire (erysipelas) and infections of the intestinal tract. Shrewsbury maintains that plague altered this picture by creating a single maximum peak in August, September and October. This new peak did not eliminate the other two because people still died of those same diseases: thus deaths at any period consisted of these plus plague. There seems to be a tendency to assume that all deaths in 1348–9 were due to plague and a true estimate of deaths resulting from the new epidemic should be the total deaths less the normal pre-plague number for the month. Despite what Shrewsbury says about the creation of a single peak in August, September and October this fact does not emerge from the Institutions to vacant benefices in the several dioceses, all vacancies being generally but probably erroneously attributed to plague deaths.

In the diocese of Salisbury the increase in Institutions begins in November 1348 rising from five in October to about 17. December, January and February 1349 are fairly constant at around 30 each but there is a peak of 60 in March which falls to just over 20 in April and in May returns to the 30 mark. There is, therefore, a high replacement rate from November to May which, if plague was present, would be unlikely to be bubonic in a temperate climate. In the following account of the time of year when the epidemic was at its peak I have used the graphs of Institutions to vacant benefices in Shrewsbury (1971). This information was taken from Lunn (1937)[4] who points out that as March was the month with the maximum Institutions in the diocese of Salisbury, the epidemic probably reached its peak in February. If this is so and there was a lag between peak mortality and the record of replacements then the peak months should all be advanced by one month, e.g. March to February and so on.

In Hereford diocese the Institutions increase steadily from one a month in January 1349 to ten a month in May and June of the same year, go up to a peak of over 30 in July and decline regularly to the January level by December 1349. The actual peak of deaths may therefore have been in the month before the peak, i.e. June, in the same way that in the diocese of Salisbury the death peak might have been February. The Worcester peak months were May, June, July and August, different again from Hereford. In Bath and Wells the vacancies appeared earlier and, beginning in December 1348 and going through to April 1349, were high. On their own they suggest that the epidemic appeared earlier in that diocese than elsewhere. It would be interesting to see comparable figures for the same time of year in the pre-plague years for all diseases as well as for those years when there were known 'epidemics' but not of 'plague'. Epidemics, of which there were many even in

TABLE 2

Institutions of clergy in the dioceses of Lincoln and York, April 1349–March 1350.

	Apr.	May	June	July.	Aug.	Sept.	Oct.	Nov.	Dec.	Jan.	Feb.	Mar.
South part of Lincoln diocese (Archdeaconries of Bedford, Buckingham, Huntingdon, Leicester, Northampton and Oxford)	12	37	83	138	95	38	23	19	11	10	10	4
North part of Lincoln diocese (Archdeaconries of Lincoln and Stow)	1	6	28	99	88	46	25	21	11	10	8	3
York diocese	1	1	7	24	37	63	51	15	18	6	9	4

pre-plague times, might have been equally severe on priests.

In the diocese of Exeter the initial increase in Institutions took place in January 1349, but the highest rate occurred from March to July inclusive. Throughout the other dioceses the peak periods of Institutions were as follows:

Norwich — May to November 1349 with the two highest months July and August. Institutions in this diocese were very high compared with the pre-epidemic month.

Ely — June and July were the peak months although, as with other dioceses, there is insufficient information both before and after the epidemic period.

Winchester — Beginning in January 1349 the number rose sharply and the three peak months were March, April and May, especially the latter two.

Lichfield — In this diocese the disease became evident in April 1349 and Institutions reached a peak in the months of July and August, declining by November to a low level.

A detailed account of the epidemic in the diocese of Lincoln by Thompson (1911) has provided some useful information on the distribution of deaths both spatially and temporally within the area. Considered with the information from the diocese of York it can be seen that in the southern deaneries of Lincoln the peak months for deaths were June, July and August 1349 (Table 2 and Fig. 5), for the deaneries of Lincoln and Stow to the north, July and August but with September quite high and in the diocese of York,

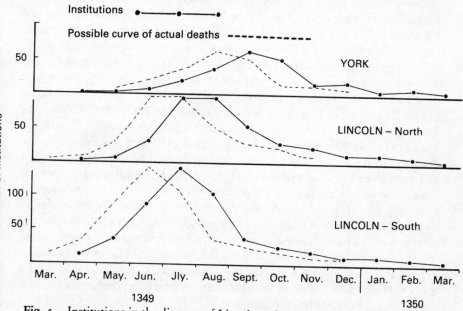

Fig. 5. Institutions in the dioceses of Lincoln and York, April 1349–March 1350

August, September and October, particularly the two latter, being the peak period. There is a suggestion here of a progression of the disease from south to north.

In the case of plague, the time of year when outbreaks occur is important because of the close relationship between flea breeding and the local climate. One would expect to predict, and plague epidemics in the current pandemic have generally been very predictable, that plague peaks would occur at roughly the same time across an area which was climatically uniform. Yet, as the Institutions show, the record of 1348–9 in England shows plague peaks at quite different times in different parts of the country. Because this does not fit the pattern for typical bubonic plague there has always been the temptation to explain this anomaly by postulating pneumonic plague as the alternative. However, outbreaks of pneumonic plague have never swept across a region in this way and the recent history of pneumonic plague in the British Isles and elsewhere, e.g. Egypt, India and South Africa (Chapter 9), does not provide adequate evidence to support the hypothesis. In fact it does quite the reverse and encourages the conviction that some other disease agent was at work.

In southern Europe the disease likewise occurred in epidemic proportions in a pattern atypical of bubonic plague for, whereas in Siena it raged from April to October 1348, Orvieto May to September 1348 and Rimini May to December 1348, in Catania it was active from October 1347 to April 1348.

It is clear, if Institutions are a true measure of the death rate, that the disease was killing many people. In the diocese of Lincoln the Institutions to benefices for the period 25 March 1349 to 24 March 1350 numbered 825, whereas the Institutions during the previous 18 months numbered 134 and in the nine months following, only 41. The latter figure is presumably so low because there were either few priests left to take up the vacancies or few willing to risk it. It should also be noted that Institutions during plague years may be inflated because resignations were more numerous during those times.

Thompson observes that the highest percentage of replacements, and presumably deaths, in the southern parts of the diocese, were generally seen in hilly and remote districts and in the neighbourhood of some of the larger towns. However, this pattern was not consistent for in the Thamesside deanery of Wycombe there was a 60 per cent replacement rate whilst Henley had only 25, yet Wendover on high ground had a mortality of 20 per cent. The deanery of Wycombe was not entirely low-lying, only the southern part along the river being so whilst to the north there was high ground. Average figures for whole deaneries, which have on some occasions considerable geographical variation as well as other points of variation, are probably misleading. Thompson's comments on a high replacement rate in the two extremes of towns on the one hand and hilly, remote areas on the other make it difficult to imagine bubonic plague as the causative disease in both cases, as my observations on rats and fleas will later show. There is no reason why more than one disease should not have been operating and this would confuse conclusions based solely on geography.

There is no really high ground in the diocese although the Chilterns provide a good contrast to the flat plain in the northern part of the diocese. There again, the general thesis related to altitude is not upheld, for the low-lying archdeaconries of Lincoln and Stow have high replacements of 44.8 per cent and 57.1 per cent respectively whilst in St Ives the losses were 23 per cent, in Holland 24 per cent and Peterborough 27 per cent. Thompson concludes that Lincolnshire, particularly north Lincolnshire, was the chief centre of the mortality in the diocese.

An important factor in the degree of mortality experienced may have been the density of the human population and perhaps also the numbers of farm animals and the type of agriculture practised. From what I shall have to say in Chapter 11 an investigation into the relationship of mortality and land usage might prove to be of greater value than other comparisons. I shall return to this theme when we come to consider the clinical nature of the disease which is believed to have caused such heavy mortality in the British Isles. Suffice to say that the spread of the epidemic continued across the country although its effect was to some extent uneven.

In some places the effect of the disease was no doubt severe. For example, in Essex (Fisher, 1943) the records from the courts of the manor of Fingreth show that at the Whit Monday court of 1348 there had been one recent death and two had occurred during the year just past. At the next court in December 1348 there was one more death but by the time the court met in late March 1349 the epidemic had arrived and 12 deaths were recorded. The court next met on 1 June 1349 when 15 deaths were reported since the last court although the claims for admission to tenements and the long list of vacant holdings taken into the lord's land indicated that 55 tenants had recently died. By 30 June 1349 a further six or seven tenants had died and by August 1349 there was one additional death. During the first six months of 1349 at least 70 tenants of the manor died: the deaths of wives and children, who were not themselves holders of property, are not recorded nor is any notice taken of the demesne servants. This figure seems rather high in the light of a statement earlier in Fisher's account where the number of tenants in 1348 was estimated to be between 60 and 65. In the record of the Court Rolls of Colchester, the year 1348–9 is recorded as 'the year of the first pestilence' (in *prima pestilencia*) and 110 wills were recorded. In 1349–50, 25 wills are recorded.

The interesting feature of this account is the fact that the peak period of plague deaths was in the period between March and June (although there had been some deaths between December 1348 and March 1349), a time of year when one would not expect the death rate to increase but perhaps even to decline (see Figure 17 for the period 1340–47). The high mortality in late spring and early summer would not be typical of bubonic plague and illustrates the point that the disease produced heavy loss of life when it first made contact in a new area, no matter what time of year that was. Even if actual bubonic plague was present it seems likely that most deaths occurring were credited to the plague and even the deaths of farm animals too. Knighton recorded that sheep died of the plague with 5000 dead in grassland, their bodies being so corrupted by the plague that neither beast nor bird would touch them. There is no evidence that plague attacks sheep and it is likely that an animal disease was probably responsible for some cattle and sheep 'murrains'.

Some scholars have maintained that the effects of the epidemic have been exaggerated. Levett (1916) who studied in some detail the effects of the Black Death on the estates of the See of Winchester pointed out that one striking fact was that the accounts were continued without a break or a change in form. Other authors had formed the impression that the changes wrought on the social pattern by the disease were far reaching. Gasquet (1908) considered that the most striking and immediate effect of the mortality was to bring about nothing less than a complete social revolution whilst Cunningham observed that it seemed as if the agriculture of the country was ruined. Levett, though, was of a different opinion and was emphatic that no one who had looked through one of the Winchester Account Rolls for 1349 or 1350 and had compared it with a similar roll ten years earlier or later could possibly support either of these statements. She maintained that a strong impression of continuity in method and prosperity was left on one's mind after a cursory examination, and that the more closely one compared details the more fully was the impression borne out. Levett concluded that about 33 per cent of the population died but pointed out that little is gained by making out an *average* death rate. The mortality in her study varied widely, not only from manor to manor but from tithing to tithing. This is an interesting point in any consideration of the spread of the epidemic and it suggests some irregular distribution of a factor or factors involved in transmission. Because of the partial and irregular character of the plague Levett draws attention to the fact that conclusions drawn from the manors contained in the Winchester Pipe Roll may justly be confronted with dissimilar evidence from other groups of manors or from other districts.

Miss Levett's conclusions (that because holdings left vacant after the Black Death were soon re-let indicated that there was little decline in settlements and population) have been challenged by Postan (1973). He points out that her study was restricted to highly profitable manors in Hampshire, Wiltshire and Somerset and excluded less profitable estates to the north. The profits were sufficiently high to maintain these estates more or less intact throughout the crisis period.

It is worth emphasising that the Black Death has dominated the study of the middle of the fourteenth century to such an extent that it has been seen as the one great sickness responsible on its own for the fall in population numbers. However, the earlier estimates of a death rate of one- to two-thirds of the population through plague (Seebohm, 1865; Gasquet, 1908) have been reviewed and modern work shows that the population had begun to decline before 1348 and that the plague losses in 1348–50 were perhaps nearer 20 per cent of the population (Russell, 1948). Baker (1973) has looked at changes in the later Middle Ages and points out that by about 1330 growth had ceased and the population was possibly declining.

On some Winchester manors years of harvest failure and summer epidemics brought exceptionally high death rates (Postan and Titow, 1958–9). They estimated death rates of 40/1000 for the whole period they studied, 1245–1347, with a rate of 52/1000 for the period of most reliable data, namely 1292–1347. As they point out, this was exceptionally high compared with many modern estimates, as the following shows:

Crude death rate in post-war England and Wales	c. 12/1000	
England in 1801	c. 25/1000	
Europe early nineteenth century	32/1000	
Sweden early nineteenth century	26–28/1000	
India 1881–1901	>41/1000	} More recent
India 1901–1921	40–50/1000	estimate
India 1890–1930	>35/1000	
India in 1930s	25/1000	
Russia in 1860s	>38/1000	
Russia in second half nineteenth century	30/1000	

The Winchester figures are confined to adults, and omit deaths of infants and small children whose mortality in pre-industrial societies was high. In Russia between 1908 and 1910 more than two-thirds of the male deaths were those of males of 20 and under and mainly those of infants and children under five. Applying the differential death rates of the Russian adult population to convert the Winchester death rates of adults into those of the population as a whole, a crude rate of 70–75/1000 would result. They conclude, therefore, that the mortality on the Winchester manors in the second half of the thirteenth and the first half of the fourteenth centuries was as high as and perhaps much higher than that in any other pre-industrial society studied.

In a population which was balanced on the edge of subsistence the effects of poor harvests were severe and in at least 34 and possibly 54 of the 83 years over a period of 110 years the high mortality was due to harvest failure. In at least six years summer epidemics were the cause e.g. 1288–9. The year of 1288 was dry with an abundant harvest and cheap bread. The summer drought was continuous and the heat intense. It is presumed that in an era of poor water supplies and primitive sanitation the wells and streams dried up. Refuse was therefore less likely to be washed away and people would drink infected water, the resultant epidemics being probably gastro-intestinal in character.

On these five Winchester manors the figures for heriots suggest a death rate for 1348–9 of near 500/1000. The authors say that the actual death rates during the epidemic may have been higher than is commonly assumed but their data cannot be employed to measure them. They point out that their survey looked at a group which was not a demographic entity but a tenurial one renewed not by births but by accessions to tenures. Thus it was possible in times of trouble for the same holding to be re-let to successive tenants in the course of a year.

The mortality in the years 1348–9 has frequently been exaggerated and treated as though no other epidemic periods could be compared to it. Serious though it undoubtedly was there is some evidence that other periods had a high death rate. Russell (1966) maintained that the pestilence and famine of 1315–17 were probably the causes of the worst catastrophe in the period between the 'Black Death' of the sixth century and 1348. He says that data from the peasants on manors of the See of Winchester show a 25 per cent higher mortality than normal for the decade 1310–19. Russell considered this pestilence to have been bacillary dysentery. In Bruges and Ypres in 1316 it was a spring and summer epidemic as it also was in England in 1322, 1323 and 1324, years of high mortality. With the plethora of diseases at the time the assumption that high death rates in winter, spring and early summer always indicated the presence of pneumonic plague is unrealistic and emphasizes the fact that once plague was believed to be present it was a convenient vehicle to explain any unusually high death rates.

Russell (1966) considered that the pneumonic form did not produce as high a death rate as the bubonic form transmitted by rats and fleas. However, even if plague was actually present there is insufficient evidence for us to separate the two forms of plague in the fourteenth century and therefore there can be no basis for a comparison of death rates from both types. Russell summarised his demographic analysis of the plague of 1348–9 by estimating a population reduction of 40 to 50 per cent (outside dry areas) by 1385, although others may not entirely agree with him and would prefer a lower figure. Hatcher (1977) considered that the estimate produced by Kosminsky (1955) of a national death rate of 30 to 45 per cent is the most reasonable one.

It is of course impossible to make any attempt at separating deaths from so-called plague from those caused by other diseases. Yet as the many and varied symptoms recorded during the Pestilence reflect the presence of a variety of infectious and other diseases, the 20 per cent reduction of the population must include these and cannot be attributed to plague alone. It is not beyond the bounds of possibility that more than one new and exceptionally virulent disease organism invaded Europe during this period.

Gottfried (1978) suggested that plague became endemic in England and that this better explained the recurrent nature of the disease than the suggestion that plague was continually reintroduced. Although he agreed with Shrewsbury that many diseases other than plague were present he was certain that evidence from the fifteenth century indicated that plague was the primary element controlling mortality in East Anglia from 1430 to 1480.

One point on which most historians are in agreement is the relatively small part played by the disease in the desertion of villages. In no part of England is there evidence of the Black Death completely emptying many villages although the reduction in population reduced many villages in size. In Norfolk (Allison, 1955–7), the desertion of villages did not begin until almost 100 years after 1348–9 and the bulk of the desertions took place in the latter half of the fifteenth century. According to that author the indirect effect of the plague was that it accentuated the economic conditions which led to the Yorkist and Tudor enclosure movement and its resultant depopulation of villages. Beresford (1954) says that in general the plague has been given too much blame for destruction of villages, and many sheep-enclosures passed by unnoticed as long as the Black Death could be invoked as an explanation.

One authentic case of a village depopulated by the Great Pestilence is that of Tusmore in Oxfordshire (Beresford and Hurst, 1971). In 1358 its lord was allowed to turn the fields into a park because every villein was dead and the Exchequer was obliged to admit that there were no taxpayers left. Another Oxford village, Tilgardesle, was similarly depopulated by the epidemic but its site still remains unlocated.

Allison, Beresford and Hurst (1965) state that there is some evidence that the population of medieval England had reached its peak at the beginning of the fourteenth century and that some settlement near the margins of cultivation was already proving untenable. According to these authors, neither the pre- nor post-plague contraction resulted in any wholesale disappearance of settlements. In Oxfordshire the periods of desertion and the certain and conjectured desertions were as follows:

	Certain desertions	Conjectured desertions
Mentioned only in Domesday Book, 1086	1	0
c. 1100–c. 1350	5	3
c. 1350–c. 1450	8	17
c. 1450–c. 1700	23	17
After c. 1700	3	0

Around 2000 villages were deserted in England during this period. Some areas suffered more than others and it has been said that this was because the plague was especially violent there. In fact the massive depopulations were uneven because of the type of countryside and agriculture. Two types of countryside had relative immunity from depopulation: areas of poor, often dry soils, where extensive woodland survived even after the thirteenth-century colonisation, e.g. Sherwood, the Weald, Arden and the Essex woodlands; and villages in the fenland, where efficient mixed agriculture thrived.

The effects of the disease demanded action of various sorts to aid the stricken communities and, equally importantly, to protect those whom the infection had not reached. Since no one knew what the disease was nor what caused it the remedies were diverse and even merciless. For example in Milan when the first cases appeared, three houses, the foci, were locked up and walled in with their inhabitants isolated and closely guarded. Many authorities were concerned with the depths of graves in which plague victims were buried. These were made broad and deep and such plague-pits have been found in many places such as Avignon and Cambridge. In the latter city the work on the foundations for the New Divinity School in Trinity Street unearthed a pit filled with skeletons which had been thrown in without any attempt at order (Williamson, 1957).

Venesection (bleeding to unconsciousness), cleansing the air by great fires, purgatives, the enjoyment of fruit and good odours, and leaving the infected region as soon as possible were all extolled as remedies. The last was practised by those who could and the present long summer recess of Parliament and the universities arose partly as a means of leaving the city during the peak epidemic months. Some remedies were pleasant but outside the reach of most, e.g. leading a very moderate and abstinent life, methods promoting cheer-fulness and optimism such as surrounding one's self with beautiful objects, flowers, jewellery etc. and remaining as much as possible in gardens. Other advice was less agreeable: it was thought that attendants who took care of latrines and those serving in hospitals and heavily malodorous places were immune to plague because poison weakened, overcame and expelled poison. As a result of this, protection was sought by spending hours daily in inhaling the vapours of latrines. More practical aid came in making provision for town officials and justices of the peace to levy a special tax for the relief of the infected people.

The physicians had little to help them in their diagnosis and treatment of plague from the writings of the classical authors. Because instruction about plague was required by the clergy and other educated people to help them in their parishes and on their estates many small pamphlets on plague were written in the fourteenth and fifteenth centuries. These are known as Plague Tracts and for information on these Singer (1916) should be consulted.

The arguments concerning the effects of the disease on the social and economic life of the country are beyond the scope of this work. In general, the changes that were already beginning were probably pushed a little faster as a result of the Black Death and the four other epidemics of the fourteenth century, but as with other aspects of the disease much that was due to other causes has often been ascribed to plague.

CHAPTER FIVE

The Black rat in northern Europe

If the disease which has become known as the Black Death was bubonic plague and spread over the whole of Europe as rapidly as it did and if it was equally destructive in town and countryside, in summer and winter, then it would without any doubt have needed the presence of a numerically populous and continuously distributed population of rats to sustain it. It is true that some places experienced a higher mortality than others and a few places escaped particularly lightly but the disease nevertheless occurred over most of the British Isles.

Even allowing for some outbreaks due to the transport of fleas in merchandise, such a blanket coverage of bubonic plague must have needed rats in town and village but, more particularly, across the wide expanses of countryside between settlements. As we shall see later (Chapter 6) the climate and surroundings were both less favourable to commensal rodents than they are today so that the rodent concerned would need to be both hardy and ubiquitous.

The question that must be answered, then, is what rodent was present in such numbers over northern Europe that it could sustain a bubonic plague epidemic of the character of the one occurring during the years 1348–50. From all known plague experience there can be only two contenders, the Black and the Brown rat, both of which can begin and maintain plague in the right climatic conditions.

The Brown rat, it is generally agreed, did not arrive and colonise Europe until the early part of the eighteenth century. Heinrich (1976) however, presented a different point of view. He described a medieval bone, which is said to be the right pelvis of a Brown rat, from an excavation at Scharstorf near today's Preetz in East Holstein. The illustration purports to show the differences in shape between the excavated bone and the pelvis of a modern Black rat as well as the similarities with that of a Brown rat. In addition to this find is described the right pelvis and femur of a Brown rat from the old town of Schleswig, the animal being much smaller than the Scharstorf rat. Fusion of the epiphyses had not taken place.[5] The author comments that the much smaller size compared with the same bones of recent times and with the Scharstorf find enables us to assume that these are the remains of a young female.

This analysis deserves some consideration. In a detailed study of the pelvis in *British Muridae and Cricetidae*,[6] J. C. Brown and I described the anatomical characteristics of many species and erected an identification key (Brown and Twigg, 1969). In our description of *Rattus rattus* and *Rattus norvegicus* we stated that 'no points of distinciton between these two species have been noted'. In our opinion it is not possible to separate them on the structure of the pelvis. Our study further examined sexual dimorphism in rats and again we came to the conclusion that it was not possible to identify the male from the female pelvis. It would thus be unlikely that one could state that the remains were of one sex or the other, especially in the case of young animals whose pelves have less differences than those of adult rodents. This material, then, is unconvincing as evidence for the presence of the Brown rat in medieval times in Schleswig-Holstein.

Heinrich dates the Preetz bones to the ninth or tenth century and the Schleswig finds from the late Middle Ages (thirteenth or fourteenth century) and argues that they are therefore much older than the illustration of a rat in the Swiss naturalist Gesner's book of animals of 1553. The author says that according to several authorities this latter animal is clearly a brown rat and although this was the earliest evidence of the Brown rat in central Europe the find he describes from Preetz would prove that the species came here 500 to 600 years earlier than previously thought, in other words in the early Middle Ages.

The anatomical evidence, in my opinion, does nothing to alter current thinking about the origin of *Rattus norvegicus* in Europe and the specimens could quite easily be those of *Rattus rattus*. The most diagnostic parts of the pelvis are missing and whilst the Preetz specimen is perhaps larger than the modern Black rat pelvis figured in the paper it is not so large as the pelvis of the Brown rat.

I have not been able to examine the illustration in Gesner but, in the light of some comments on medieval illustrations of rodents in the Book of Kells (Sullivan, 1914) by Dr D. E. Davis (personal communication) who points out that in old pictures various kinds of rodents look alike, care should be taken in these identifications. Even if Gesner depicted what looked like a Brown rat he could have travelled in Russia or further East and either seen the Brown rat in its area of origin or copied the animal from illustrations elsewhere.

The Black rat is thought to have been the species that was responsible for carrying plague in Europe in the Black Death and during the next three hundred years when outbreaks are believed to have occurred at fairly regular intervals. Several writers have stated their opinions as to when this rat arrived in Britain and many more have written extensively about plague with the assumption that the Black rat was involved. The attitude to the biology of rats in the British Isles in the Middle Ages can be summed up in this way; there was bubonic plague, therefore there must have been rats.

R. S. R. Fitter (1959), calling the species 'the old English black rat', says that it is not known when it arrived in the British Isles and that it does not seem to have been recorded with certainty anywhere in western Europe before the twelfth or thirteenth century. The Crusades took place during the period 1095–1229 and it has been generally assumed that the first rats arrived with the returning Crusaders. But, as Fitter says, there is no positive evidence that rats came back with them and if they did it is odd that no contemporary clues have come down in legend or folk names linking rats with the Crusaders. On the other hand, Fitter says that rats were probably present in late twelfth-century Britain.

Giraldus Cambrensis tells how the larger mice that were commonly called rats (qui vulgariter rati vocantur) were expelled from Fernegenal (in Ireland) by the bishop, St Yvor, whose books they had eaten. As a result of this, he says, there were no more indigenous rats remaining nor did introduced stock succeed in establishing itself. Before taking even the presence of rats too literally one should bear in mind that Giraldus describes how St Patrick expelled venomous reptiles from the whole of Ireland, whereas the truth of the matter is that they never succeeded in entering the country. It is also said that in Wales a Welshman was eaten by rats. However, there may have been some discrepancy in the reporting of this event. Giraldus tells how in the province of Cemmeis a young man had a severe illness during which he suffered a violent persecution from toads which came in great numbers to him. His nurses and friends destroyed as many as they could but they made little effect on their numbers and in desperation tied the man in a bag and hoisted him to the top of a high tree which they stripped of its leaves. Sadly, he was not secure even there for the toads crept up the tree in great numbers and consumed him even to his very bones. He concludes 'It is also recorded that by the hidden but never unjust will of God another man suffered a similar persecution from rats' (Everyman edition, 1908). As Prys-Jones (1955) points out, Giraldus fails to inform us whether they gobbled him up in the end or not.

Barrett-Hamilton (1913) states that there is little doubt that the Black rat came to Europe in the navies of the Crusaders and that whilst it was firmly established in western Europe shortly afterwards, there was no clear evidence of its presence prior to the Crusades of 1095, 1147 and 1191.

Russell (1968), pointing out that in Britain a pattern of plague periodicity existed similar to that seen in the sixth- and seventh-century plagues, considered that this identity of pattern suggests that the rat was present, since no other rodent quite fills the place. Hirst (1953) has some very positive things to say in support of the presence of the Black rat in northern Europe in early times but presents little in the way of evidence. He regards the view that rats were scarce in the British Isles during the fourteenth century as quite untenable and considers it probable that true rats were well known in Anglo-Saxon England, having been probably brought over by Anglo-Saxon invaders from Germanic lands. He considers that at the time of the Black Death in 1348–50, during the plague of London and continental cities and later until the Brown rat came to Europe at the beginning of the eighteenth century, the Black rat must have been present in sufficient numbers to cause serious epidemics, providing it carried enough fleas capable of transmitting plague to man. He further considers that a swarming of Black rats might have begun the great epidemic.

Macfarlane Burnet (1962) considered that one of the most important determining factors in the plague of 1348 was the thirteenth-century spread to Europe of the Black rat, *Mus rattus* (=*Rattus rattus*), a native of India which reached Europe with the returning Crusaders. There '*it rapidly replaced indigenous rats* and flourished in and around human habitations'. There were no indigenous rats, of course, and this is a surprising statement for an eminent authority on disease.

Recent writers have provided a wealth of unwarranted supposition on the topic of the Black rat. Going back to Issyk Koul, Ziegler (1970) says that the tarbagan, jerboa and suslik *probably* were present there and also the rat, although its main role was not to come till the disease was on the move. He then compounds this by saying that in order to disturb the quiet and generally harmless existence of *Pasteurella pestis*[7] something had to happen to make the rodents leave their homes. There is no reason to postulate this because all evidence on plague spread in both murine and sylvatic phases suggests that plague spreads through a population of rodents by contact with fleas. There is no evidence to support rodent migration as a factor in plague spread and only a very few authenticated cases of rodents leaving an area *en masse* because of some calamity such as fire or flood.

There is, however, some slight evidence that on a local basis plague may be influenced by agricultural flooding practices. In Madagascar there was a distinct parallel between the frequency and subsidence of plague and the alternating flooding and draining of the rice fields. On the plateau the rats (*R. r. alexandrinus*) left the villages during the dry season to settle down in the fields, and returned to the settlements when the flooding of the plantations began. Spring floods have been shown to be a major means of population reduction of *Rattus norvegicus* in Ohio as the rats fled from flooded cornfields and became easy prey (Chapman, 1938).

Ziegler says that we are unlikely ever to know exactly what it was which caused this particular rodent migration, but that such evidence as survives (it would be interesting to know the nature of this evidence) suggests that they were driven away by floods, although on other occasions prolonged droughts have caused emigration, or that the population became too large for the available food supply. I have not been able to find any authenticated accounts of rodent emigration resulting from drought. Those rodents which live in habitats where droughts occur seem able to exist quite well on the water stored in seeds and roots and, furthermore, have certain physiological mechanisms for retaining body water by reducing its loss in urine. Likewise, rodents adapt their rate of population increase and their density to ensure that overpopulation of resources is largely avoided. Studies on field rodents such as voles, which regularly produce large numbers, have shown that the percentage of available food energy consumed per year is on average 7.8.

Ziegler considers that not only did a massive exodus take place but that it was above all *Rattus rattus*, which he calls 'the tough, nimble, by nature vagabond, black rat', which made the move. *Rattus rattus* is, though, essentially sedentary, moves little under any provocation and, in any case, there is no written record of any such movement. Even if there was a record it is highly improbable that the Black rat could be identified either by the chroniclers of the time or even by modern scholars from contemporary accounts.

Shrewsbury (1971) contradicts Ziegler when he comments that there does not appear to be any record of the House rat (*Rattus rattus*) ever having been seen crossing even a small river, and that *as it is not normally a migratory animal* it does not usually move far from its birthplace of its own accord. He considered, though, that it may be forced to emigrate by the stress of famine or the goad of an epizootic disease such as plague. He is correct in assessing its sedentary nature but there is no evidence at all that rats move under the stress of an epizootic. They die in the houses in which they live and in their holes within these buildings.

The topic of migration, a term incorrectly used for a mass movement of rats, is probably one which generates more inaccurate comments than most other aspects of rodent life. Shrewsbury says that *Rattus norvegicus* is normally shy of man and in temperate climates will not breed in close contact with him. This is not entirely true as the Brown rat will breed in close proximity to man and his activities, for example in coal mines (Twigg, 1975). He also says that, 'It is naturally a migratory animal, performing a partial migration at different seasons, sometimes travelling long distances when seized by the migratory impulse and crossing wide rivers, deserts and mountainous regions in the course of its migrations'. This has no substance in fact and a study of the spread of the species in North America shows quite the opposite. The Brown rat has edged steadily across the cultivated regions but deserts and mountains have proved a barrier to its progress unless transported in merchandise across the inhospitable regions.

Russell (1968) adds further to the confused thinking about rats and plague when he compares the plague of Justinian with the fourteenth-century outbreak. Noting that there was some similarity in periodicity in the two periods he claimed that, 'the reason seems to be the periodic expansion of the rat population which carried it far beyond the normal limits of its range'. If, however, plague had already covered the British Isles, and presumably rats similarly existed over the whole area to account for the disease, then it is difficult to see how periodic outbreaks could have anything to do with rats expanding their range since they were already there. What he probably had in mind was the periodic recrudescence of existing foci but this is a different matter altogether.

Russell (1966) suggests that the plague epidemics may follow the cycle of rodent expansion of about 3.86 years but this figure applies only to certain rodents such as lemmings and voles (Wing, 1957, 1961). There is no evidence that rats have any such cyclic component in their biology.

It is unlikely that we shall ever be able to have incontrovertible evidence as to whether *Rattus rattus* was present in Britain, or indeed northern Europe, on a wide scale. Isolated records of Black rat remains are recovered from time to time in archaeological sites and are used as evidence but such recoveries must be carefully assessed. The Black rat in temperate latitudes today lives only in the warmer parts of towns and it is likely that it has always done so. Some rats must inevitably have been carried in merchandise and some buildings of ports and cities would probably have been warm enough to enable local populations to survive and maintain themselves without regular importation of fresh stock.

Rackham (1979) has reported the finding of rodent skeletal material claimed to be that of at least two specimens of *Rattus rattus* from the lower part of a Roman well constructed in the late second or third century in York and thought to have been in use until the late fourth century A.D. The author excludes the possibility that the rats had entered either as live animals or skeletal elements into the backfill of the well after its deposition. He considers that the close set timbers lining the well and the hard clay and cobble packing in the construction shaft would have prevented any possible entry from the sides. The excavators were of the opinion that there were no burrows or gaps in the fill which would have allowed rats to penetrate down through five metres of deposit. These points, together with the fact that the habits of the Black rat are such that it is said to avoid burrowing to any depth in a damp soil, were all considered evidence against the rats entering the well after backfilling. The conclusion that the specimens were at least pre-eighth century would push back the date of the introduction of the Black rat into Britain by about four hundred years.

Rackham reviews the various claims for the presence of *Rattus rattus* in Britain and finds little direct evidence for the occurrence of this rat in the British Isles before the fourteenth century other than the specimens he describes and the remains of seven 'rats' from the period 1250–1350 recovered from excavations in medieval Southampton (Noddle, 1975). No details of species are available for the latter specimens but it must be assumed that they were *Rattus rattus*. There is now archaeological evidence for the presence of a probable Black rat in tenth-century A.D. London (Armitage, 1979) and Black rat remains from the Baynard's Castle site in fourteenth-century London

(Armitage, 1977) as well as from third- and fourth-century A.D. London (Armitage *et al.*, 1984).

We can learn much about the distribution of small mammals from the way in which their remains are present in the residues of the food of certain predators, notably owls. These birds swallow rodents more or less intact, having no teeth with which to chew them, and having digested the soft parts regurgitate the bones and hair in the form of a compacted pellet. From this pellet the skulls, teeth and other bones are easily identified and it is possible to build up a picture of the species taken by an owl in any habitat.

In the countryside in Britain today the pellets of the Barn owl regularly contain remains of Brown rat, especially where the owl has hunted over farmland and around farm buildings. If, therefore, as is frequently suggested, *Rattus rattus* had been present in the Middle Ages its remains should have appeared in pellets. However, Dr T. P. O'Connor has carried out some interesting work on this aspect of medieval biology and has very kindly allowed me to quote from his unpublished results. He found owl pellets from early thirteenth-century levels at Caerleon, near Newport, Gwent, in Wales. A Roman *frigidarium* which was still a substantial ruin in the thirteenth century had been colonised by owls for a long time with the result that a very large deposit of small mammal bones, probably representing as many as 100,000 individuals, had accumulated. From the prey species he considered that the Barn owl had been the hunter and although many species of small mammal, including the house mouse, were present there were no rats. This is important evidence and the absence of a rural rat population is a strong argument against the presence of a widespread rat population and extensive epizootic plague. It might be argued that because the Black rat would be confined to buildings then its chances of being taken by a barn owl would be remote. If that is so then it still rules out the presence of an epizootic linking one habitation with the next.

The Black rat has been reported from Lincoln (O'Connor, 1982). Three specimens were recovered from the Flaxengate site. One was dated to the later ninth century (probably about 860–880), one to 900–930 and the third to about 1040–60/70, i.e. just pre-Norman.

Discussing the available evidence for the presence of the Black rat, Rackham refers to a statement attributed to Hirst (1953) that epidemics only arise in urban situations when rats are present, and that the disease is only sustained under these conditions when the rat population is well established. He therefore concludes from this that to plot the distribution of historic occurrences of bubonic plague will serve as an indirect means of plotting the ancient distribution of the Black rat.

If we could be certain that the epidemics were bubonic plague this would be a good approach. However, another way of looking at this question of whether the Black rat was present on a wide scale is to examine the nature of the environment in the Middle Ages and to compare it with those environments where the Black rat is successful today. That might be more instructive than arguing whether isolated finds are indicative of the widespread presence of rats.

The standard texts on plague such as Hirst (1953), Pollitzer (1954) and Shrewsbury (1971) are all agreed that rats were present. Dr David E. Davis has written a paper which may be published before my research is presented in which he outlines his scepticism about the presence of *Rattus rattus* during the Black Death and he has very kindly allowed me to draw on his findings in this account. On some of his points I differ but in general I support his thesis although from a different angle.

As he points out, some writers have produced very solid numbers for medieval times e.g. Ziegler, who says that the norm was one rat family per household and three fleas per rat. Russell (1968) also produces some extraordinarily precise figures and some curious ecological information in his comments on plague in England in 1348–50. He says that a rat's territory was apparently a house or even an apartment house (2.3 rats to each in India) and there were on the average 3.7 fleas to the rat. It is difficult enough to acquire such precise information from modern times on these two points (Davis, 1953a) and quite impossible from medieval times. Rat or flea numbers in English houses in 1349 cannot be assumed from data acquired in Indian dwellings in 1910.

Davis observes that great reliance in support of the view that rats were present has been placed on old pictures but, as he points out, the rodents illustrated in the Book of Kells which have been called rats by Shrewsbury, could be any one of several native species. MacArthur (1957) considered that the rodents in the Book of Kells were rats with the external characters of *Rattus rattus*. However, Armitage (1977) questions this identification and, whilst agreeing that the animals are rodent-like, points out that there is insufficient detail to enable them to be positively identified as Black rats. All the animals are highly stylised and cats and rodents may not have been drawn to the same scale: if the scales are different then the rodents could be mice and not rats. After looking carefully at these rodents nibbling the Eucharistic bread I tend to agree with Armitage.

Davis considers that in the absence of both Black and Brown rat the Water vole, *Arvicola amphibius*, would have been noticed by rural and even urban people, although in view of the inability of medieval people to furnish precise descriptions one must feel dubious about such a capability. Another point is that evidence about rodent species may be available in comments about cats in medieval literature. Davis says that cats have difficulty with large *Rattus* and catch only small ones. He considers that they find *Arvicola* and *Microtus* easy prey and capture many. Certainly *Microtus* is easy, being quite small, but it would be interesting to know just how easy would be a large specimen of *Arvicola*, which could weigh upwards of 300 g (Southern, 1964).

Davis considers that the illustrations in the Book of Kells probably represent *Arvicola*. In Shrewsbury (1971) there is a picture depicting rodents hanging a cat. These are large animals but their tails are only half the length of the head and body, a feature more indicative of *Arvicola* than *Rattus*. From the illustrations in four bestiaries produced from 1121 to 1218 there were no pictures of rats, nor in the pictures of 739 animals from illuminated Gothic manuscripts. About 70 kinds of animals were mentioned but no rats.

In a translation of a twelfth-century Latin bestiary (White, 1954) is an illustration of *Mus*, the mouse. This animal is neither rat- nor mouse-like. The head is roughly rodent-like but the body is very chubby and the tail very pointed with a thick base and is much shorter than the length of head and body. Attempts at determining any precise identification of animals like rats and mice, not always easy today, from medieval bestiaries should be viewed with extreme caution because it was not considered important at the time to make accurate likenesses.

On the question of written evidence Davis comments that it seems clear that travellers knew rats from the Middle East because there is a picture of a rat in Persia in 1291. In addition he says that Campbell (1931) examined 70 tracts written before 1400 on the topic of the Black Death, none of which mentions rats, and that Coulton (1930) found no mention of the rat in 922 pages of translated documents. There is, however, a reference to rats in Holland in Volume IV of Coulton where St Lydwine of Schiedam (1380–1433), suffering from severe ulcers, beseeched the parson for capon fat to put on a plaster for her sores. When he refused, saying that the capons he had killed were very thin, she exclaimed, 'God grant that they may all be eaten of rats', a curse which was immediately fulfilled. Later, the same lady asked the priest for some apples and he, remembering what had befallen the capons, said, 'I will give the girl a few, lest they be eaten of dormice'.

In Piers Plowman is the well-known account of belling the cat. Text B (ed. Davis, J. F.) refers to 'ratones at ones, And small mys myd hem', ratones being translated as small rats. The editor observes that this was a well-known fable, the earliest forms being found in a Latin collection of Odo de Cheriton in the thirteenth century and Skeat (1962) has listed several occurrences of this fable. It would be interesting to know exactly where it had its origins. Davis (D. E.) comes to the conclusion that a search of the literature of the past does not produce any real evidence of rats in fourteenth-century Europe.

It has been argued that a clear warning of impending plague would be given by the conspicuous mortality of rats which occurs in the epizootic and that this would have been noted and recorded by contemporary writers. I can find none recorded and in other epidemics such as the one documented by Cipolla (1973) there has been a failure to note rat deaths. Cipolla describes the plague of 1630 in northern Italy and quotes from an anonymous writer who described the course of plague in the small town of Busto Arsizio between Como and Milan and had this to say about the rats:

in 1630 there prevailed such a great quantity of rats that people could hardly protect themselves either at daytime or at night from the molesting rage of these animals. Neither was it possible to save anything from their fury because of their great number. One could count them by the hundreds in every house and they were so big that people went in terror of them. They damaged everything and especially woollens and linens and they were so hungry that they gnawed at doors and windows.

It is difficult to take all this at face value. The rat species could only be *Rattus rattus*, a gentle, shy animal which is neither so large nor so fierce as to cause human fear and records from crowded houses in India (Chapter 6) have never shown large rat numbers like these per house. Despite this possible exaggeration, there is no mention of dead rats: if they were present in such density then the epizootic should have been particularly evident.

However, Campbell (1931) in a discussion of modern knowledge about plague and the part played by rats says:

> While such an origin of the disease did not become known till late in the nineteenth century and was not suspected by our medieval ancestors, it was noted by Avicenna that a sign of pestilence was when mice and animals living under the earth fled to its surface and were disturbed as if they were drunk; and observations of disturbance in the animal world are made by several fourteenth century writers.

Davis says that epidemics of plague can occur without rats and supports this by reference to Hankin (1905) who observed that in India only eight of 40 local epidemics had obvious rat mortality. Hankin, however, did not actually observe this himself and was quoting from the work of Dr Planck who, in Garhwal, had observed a phenomenon which was, in Hankin's account 'curious'. In Garhwal outbreaks of plague which were due to a proved, and recent, importation of the disease were never accompanied by a mortality among rats. When Hankin wrote, the study of plague was in its infancy and clearly the part played by rats was little understood, as evidenced by his remark that, 'rats are not a necessary cause or agent in the spread of plague'. Whatever may have been the situation in Garhwal there was never any doubt that rats were involved in Bombay, yet Hankin wrote, 'Evidence obtained during the Bombay outbreak, as also the evidence from Garhwal, leaves little room for doubt that rats are not a necessary factor in the spread of plague. In Garhwal out of forty outbreaks investigated by Planck a rat mortality was only observed in eight'. Widening his argument, Hankin compares the situation in Garhwal with the Black Death which he considers analogous for, whereas when that disease reached Constantinople it was accompanied by rat mortality, no such phenomenon was recorded during its spread through the rest of Europe.

The supposed references to a connection between rats and plague by

European medieval authors are thought for the most part to be based on the quotation from Avicenna but according to one author there was no adequate reason for believing that any noticeable rat mortality ever accompanied plague in the Middle Ages in Europe. On the other hand, Eastern authors are said not infrequently to refer to rats staggering about as if drunk in times of plague.

Whilst, in the early Indian experience and elsewhere, *obvious* rat mortality may have been absent it is no evidence that mortality was lacking. Rats die in holes and in thatched roofs without being seen and as long as their fleas can contact people there will be human cases. There must be rats, or some other rodents, from which plague proceeds in the first place and it is difficult to substantiate evidence of a bubonic plague *epidemic*, as distinct from spasmodic cases, breaking out without infected rodents being somewhere in the vicinity.

Ziegler argues this point, too, and says that though the rat helps considerably in the spread of bubonic plague, he agrees with Professor Jorge that it is not essential. He quotes from the Plague Research Commission of 1910 which pointed out that the transference of infected rats and fleas in merchandise or, in the case of fleas, on the body of a human being, must be considered. He agrees with those who have said, and Dr Hirst who has shown, that the adage of 'No ship rats, no plague' is clearly untrue and points to the fact that *Xenopsylla cheopis*, in ideal conditions, can live for a month away from its host. Such a flea, travelling with a cargo of grain or in a bale of cloth, could therefore easily travel hundreds of miles without a rat. Furthermore, he quotes a substantiated case of a flea surviving unfed for six months in a rat burrow and concludes that the absence of rats was no guarantee that bubonic plague could never occur.

It is true that one infected flea could travel in merchandise and infect a person unpacking the goods. Several fleas could cause several cases but, unless those infected fleas contact and infect the local rat population then such a series of cases will be of an isolated, local nature and will not constitute an epidemic. During this century there has been ample opportunity to see this. Transfer of plague by the human flea is rare and although in ideal conditions *X. cheopis* may live for a month without its host it is doubtful if at the end of that time it could transmit plague. As a rule, when not on a host, conditions are far from ideal and militate against the most effective transmission. The only way in which a major epidemic can start by fleas alone is in the case of transfer to the pneumonic phase when a single case with pulmonary involvement could trigger off many more. As I shall demonstrate later even the documented outbreaks of pneumonic plague have been of relatively short duration and limited in geographical extent as well as being primary pneumonic plague in a special set of climatic conditions.

As for the case of a flea surviving unfed for six months in a *rat* burrow I have not been able to find this in the literature although in blocked burrows of the African gerbil, *Tatera brantsi*, Davis (1953b) recovered plague-infected fleas of the species *X. philoxera* 120 days after the warrens became untenanted. Pirie (1927) found that infected fleas (*Dinopsyllus lypusus* and *X. eridos*) in experimental enclosures survived without a host for three and *possibly* four months and were capable of transmitting plague to 'clean' rodents (gerbilles, species not given) put into the enclosures.

If we are to arrive at any conclusions about the way the Black rat could have been effective as a plague carrier in the fourteenth century it will be necessary to examine in detail all aspects of the biology of this species. The Black rat is a native of the Indian region and came to the Mediterranean by way of Asia Minor. It or its sub-species spread north and eventually came to occupy many parts of Europe. The true Black rat appears when two forms – the dark brown *frugivorus* and the light brown *alexandrinus* – interbreed. This form, like all melanics (black forms), is hardier in a cold climate and, it is said, became the dominant form in northern Europe after the medieval invasions. The original wild form is *frugivorus*, with *alexandrinus* a darker one adapted, like the house mouse, to living in man-made shelter in cool climates and the very dark *rattus* an adaptation to even cooler climates. The species is smaller in build than the Brown rat and has a different way of life. The Brown rat is essentially a ground dweller and burrows extensively in many types of soil including wet environments. In the British Isles it is found living in hedgerows, fields, the banks of rivers and canals, on the seashore, in coal mines (Twigg, 1961) and sewers (Barnett and Bathard, 1953; Bentley, Bathard and Hammond, 1955). It extends throughout all parts of the British Isles, being found in any place, no matter how cold and wet, providing there is adequate food and shelter and has spread to most parts of the world from its central Asian source. In tropical regions it is the chief rat of the ports.

The Black rat is much more circumscribed in its choice of habitat in northern Europe and probably the chief factor influencing its selection of a living site is temperature. It is almost totally dependent upon the warmth provided by human habitations and warehouses and even when more widespread than today it was rarely found away from buildings. To quote from an old rodent control circular: 'even in countryside before the arrival of *Rattus norvegicus*, black rats always seem to have been confined to buildings and have never lived for long in hedges and fields as brown rats now do'. Bentley (1959) was also clear about this (see Chapter 6, p. 100). Some work in northern Germany has shown that whereas the Brown rat prefers a temperature of 35.06°C the Black rat selects a temperature of 38.09°C. These observations were made on 350 Brown and 300 Black rats (Herter, 1950).

It must surely be considered remarkable that the Black Death could behave with such freedom in terms of season and climate in north-west Europe and yet be so circumscribed by the impositions of climate in warm regions. The disease apparently reached the polar regions and according to Thomson (1975) it struck Greenland even more savagely than Europe. It is highly unlikely that *Rattus rattus* was present there at that time and I can find no records of this species in Greenland in modern times either. If there had been introductions they would have had to live very close to man to survive. Even the much hardier *Rattus norvegicus* finds it necessary to seek out warm human habitations in such a climate. In Alaska where the winter is harsh, with the absolute minimum January temperature −47°C (−117°F) and where days colder than −40°C (−104°F) are common, rats make every effort to find winter refuge in heated buildings with a food supply. Unsuccessful animals are frostbitten and some die of cold. As a result of the harsh conditions the population is very low by April (Schiller, 1956).

In cooler, temperate areas the Black rat tends to be restricted to ports (Corbet and Southern, 1974) and during recent time in the British Isles it has been confined solely to seaports and to those inland towns connected to the ports by canals, the rats from ships inhabiting the dockland warehouses being transported in cargoes by barge to inland towns.

Bentley (1959) showed that in Britain between 1951 and 1956 this rat had decreased in range and frequency in most localities and had disappeared from some. In 1951 it was present in 90 local authorities, many in London but others as widespread as Penzance, Lerwick and Belfast, with the main populations in Bristol, Liverpool and London. It has progressively disappeared from inland towns as the canal links with feeder ports were lost.

The distribution in London was especially interesting with rats being more widely spread than anywhere else in the United Kingdom and established in

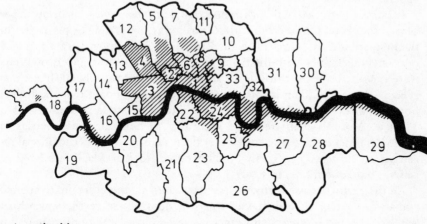

Key to authorities:

1. City of London	10. Hackney	18. Brentford & Chiswick	26. Lewisham
2. Holborn	11. Stoke Newington	19. Wandsworth	27. Greenwich
3. Westminster	12. Hampstead	20. Battersea	28. Woolwich
4. St. Marylebone	13. Paddington	21. Lambeth	29. Erith
5. St. Pancras	14. Kensington	22. Southwark	30. East Ham
6. Finsbury	15. Chelsea	23. Camberwell	31. West Ham
7. Islington	16. Fulham	24. Bermondsey	32. Poplar
8. Shoreditch	17. Hammersmith	25. Deptford	33. Stepney
9. Bethnal Green			

Fig. 6   Distribution of *R. rattus* – London 1951 (after Bentley, 1959).

all the riparian boroughs to the south of the Thames from Erith westwards to Wandsworth, except Deptford which has a very short river frontage (Fig. 6). No local authority on the south bank reported its presence very far inland, its restriction to riverside buildings being especially marked in Wandsworth, Battersea and Lambeth. North of the Thames it was a different picture. Not only was *R. rattus* present in several docks and within the boundaries of every riparian authority from West Ham westwards to Fulham (except Chelsea) but was also established through Holborn, St Marylebone, the southern half of Finsbury, Islington, Shoreditch and the south-west of Bethnal Green.

Central London, therefore, provided conditions favourable for the establishment of the rat. These were the presence of numerous, multi-storied, centrally heated and, particularly, non-residential buildings interspersed with restaurants, canteens and other food sources. Being an animal which climbs well it was ideally suited to life in the great multi-storey buildings of ports. The idea that it was driven out by the Brown rat is scarcely tenable because competition for living space between the two species is negligible. The Brown rat does not climb for choice and is content to occupy the cellars and basements. Even today in London the Black rat can be found in the upper storeys and the Brown rat in the ground floor and below. However, the need for warmth may cause the Black rat to live low down in buildings as Matheson (1939) reported in a Cardiff cinema where *Rattus norvegicus* lived in the space beneath the stage whilst *Rattus rattus* lived in the basement where the heating apparatus was located.

In tall seven-storied buildings in Bombay *Rattus norvegicus* made up 30 per cent of the ground floor catch with *Rattus rattus* comprising 65 per cent. On the first, second and third floors the Brown rat made up 19.8, 12.4 and 13.8 per cent respectively with the Black rat making up the rest. No Brown rats were caught above the third floor, all rats above that level being Black rats (Plague Research Commission, 1907). Aitken (1899) noted that the Indian house rat was a nimble climber which always took up its quarters in the roof of a house. Most lived in trees and according to him came into houses in monsoon times more than at any other time. As early as 1768 the official rat catcher to Princess Amelia in London remarked that Black rats lived in ceilings but Brown ones in sewers.

Rattus rattus is essentially a sedentary animal, therefore in temperate climates its occurrence in towns where it does not leave the warmth of buildings is a fact of great significance in the aetiology of bubonic plague and one we should remember when viewing past epidemics of that disease.

The reproductive capacity of rats in any given climate and habitat will also determine when there are high rat populations. If these coincide with the warmer times of the year, when conditions are optimal for flea breeding, we may expect plague cases to be at their maximum then. The mortality of Black rats is high and between 91 and 97 per cent of a population dies each year (Davis, 1953a). To keep pace with this the reproductive capacity must be high. In the British Isles the embryo rate[8] is recorded as 6.9 in warehouses and buildings in the Port of London and 7.5 on ships in the port (Watson, 1950), with peak breeding on shore during September. According to Watson, who examined 4131 *R. rattus* in the Port of London between September 1941 and September 1943, the breeding figures for London shore rats were similar in general to those for various Indian rat populations investigated by the Indian Plague Commission. Females have between three and five litters per year.

In some places, e.g. Cyprus, a bimodal curve of pregnancy has been noted. In parts of the world where there has been recent plague, such as India and Egypt, the breeding of the Black rat has been extensively studied. In India the reproductive curves for Belgaum, Poona, Punjab, Bengal and Bombay are generally unimodal, with minima in the cold, dry season. Belgaum and Punjab, however, showed additional pregnancy peaks in the monsoon season. In Egypt there is low reproduction in the winter.

In Czechoslovakia, Figala (1964) collected *Rattus rattus* from brick-built corn ricks, mills, poultry farms, granaries and pig stalls and examined their reproduction rates. He concluded that the small proportion of nestlings in the winter months indicated their high mortality in habitats with low temperatures, this being another cause of limitation in the reproduction of Black rats in that region.

We have little information on the density of Black rats per unit area in Europe, the nearest estimation I can find is that of two to five rats per acre (five to 12 per hectare) in Cyprus scrubland (Watson, 1951). In Freetown, Sierra Leone, in the dry season of 1937, Leslie and Davis (1939) attempted to estimate the absolute number of rats in an area of 22.5 acres. During six weeks, 630 breakback traps were set in 210 houses and they concluded that there were between 407 and 563 *R. rattus* on the area when the experiment started, i.e. between 18 and 25 rats per acre or between 1.9 and 2.7 rats per house.

In any habitat the density is likely to be related to the availability of food and shelter. For the Black rat in northern Europe buildings may have been as important in determining distribution and density in the fourteenth century as they are today and it is perhaps no chance occurrence that finds associate the species with human habitation.. Important also would be the construction of dwellings and the climate of the British Isles in the fourteenth century, factors to be considered in the next chapter.

CHAPTER SIX

The rat environment

The existence of a widely distributed Black rat population in fourteenth-century Britain would have been dependent upon certain features. Of considerable importance would be the distribution of the human population and the degree of urbanisation. As rats possibly existed in Roman settlements the degree of continuity between these and the towns of the Middle Ages must be considered.

The size of the human population and its distribution would be important as would also the size of settlements and the type of vegetation covering the country. In addition, the construction of buildings and their capacity for rat harbourage in town and village must be considered. Climate, too would be of great importance and whilst I shall mention it briefly it is better considered in the following chapter which deals with the biology of the flea.

Various estimates of the size of the human population of Britain during the mid-fourteenth century have been made by historians and demographers. Coulton (1949) said there was fairly general agreement that England and Wales had about 2.5 million at the Conquest and about five million under Henry VII. Seeing that this covers a period of 450 years during which time epidemics reduced the population and the normal reproductive processes tended to increase it, it does not help very much in trying to arrive at an immediate pre-plague figure. The problem of assessing this population is further impeded by the fact that there was no census between the Domesday Survey and the Poll Tax returns of 1377. Russell (1948) says that in 1377 the population (approximately 2.23 million) was about 60 per cent of the 1346 population. This would give a pre-plague figure of around 3.7 million and Shrewsbury (1971) suggests a figure of four million as the maximum for the 1348 population. Ziegler (1970) sums up the evidence and considers that the population could have been somewhere in the range between 3.7 million and 4.6 million and settles for a figure of 4.2 million.

Earlier estimates had been somewhat further away from modern thinking on this matter. Thorold Rogers (1866) had calculated from the amount of wheat grown that the population even at its maximum before the pestilence could have been no more than 1.5 million. Even though he was prepared to admit that it might have been as high as 2.5 million he was adamant that the rate of production of food could not have supported any more people. Bennett (1938) accepted that the 1066 population was 2.5 million and reckoned that even the most optimistic estimate for 1349 could not exceed 5.0 million.

Postan (1975) has summed up the difficulties most concisely. He pointed out that medieval England, unlike any other medieval country, possessed at least two sources capable of presenting estimates of the total population, i.e. the Domesday Book of 1086 and the Poll Tax returns of 1377. The former appears to list all the tenants of land whilst the latter purports to tax, and thus record, the entire adult population. As Postan said, with these sources available the temptation to estimate the population at these two times has been great. He believed that such estimates are unreliable because both sources do not contain true enumerations of the populace but numbers of certain sections of the population. He considered that before a true population aggregate could be derived from these numbers they should be supplemented by estimates for the missing sections; or, more precisely, they should be multiplied by coefficients representing the proportion by which the numbers fall short in the total. But even then he thought that the construction of the coefficients was fraught with such uncertainties and errors so great as to make the whole enterprise worthless.

Both Coulton (1949) and Kosminsky (1956) are in general agreement as to the proportion of the population dwelling in towns. The former considered that at least 90 per cent of the population were villagers and the latter that 12 per cent or just under lived in cities or towns. This would mean that roughly 400,000 were town dwellers leaving approximately three and a half million to be distributed amongst the villages.

Russell (1948) gives the estimated populations of the 19 major towns of England in 1377. After correcting these figures to the 1348 level by adding 40 per cent, the total comes to just over 165,000 people, leaving another 235,000 to be accounted for. There were many more towns and Heighway (1972) lists the criteria which may be used to help in the classification of a town. These are varied and include such things as urban defences, an internal street plan, a market, a mint, a diversified economic base, and several other features, the possession of which separates such communities from the villages. There were also, in addition to these economic criteria, legal ones. Using these various criteria we see that many of today's towns, including those on List IV (historic towns with no modern urban administrative status), did not exist as such in 1348. Nevertheless, in England alone there were no fewer than 662 towns by the time the epidemic arrived (there are 1109 today), many of them only achieving town status by the thirteenth century. In order to house the remaining 235,000 each so-called town would only contain approximately 350 people. This would not raise it above the level of a village for Coulton gives the average population for a village in western Europe as between 200 and 400 or 450 and containing from 40 to 80 adult males. Levett (1916) calculated that the Manor of Orchard in the See of Winchester housed about 38 households, giving a population of about 190.

The 3.5 million rural dwellers would, on the above estimates, be spread out amongst a fairly large number of villages. Platt (1978) says that there were 13,000 vills individually named in Domesday and that this number was not significantly increased, at least by permanent settlements, until very recent times. He points out that village-type settlements were not the norm everywhere in England. Many of the vills of the Domesday Survey were very small and there were areas such as Devonshire where isolated homesteads were the usual farming unit. However, the notion that there was a marked contrast between the north and west where hamlets and single farmsteads were the dominant settlement and central, eastern and southern England where compact, nucleated villages were the main unit is much too simple according to Hoskins (1977). He says that in Cornwall and Devon the large, compact village can be found all over as early as the Norman Conquest whilst very old hamlets and isolated farmsteads can be found in the midland and eastern counties. There were, therefore, many small units containing people and food but their distribution would be important in plague dissemination because of its effect upon population density in any given region.

Let us first consider the possibility that the Black rat was introduced by the Romans, as suggested by Rackham (1979), and had entered the British Isles by at least the fourth century A.D.. The Roman occupation began in A.D. 43 and ended almost 400 years later, in A.D. 409 or perhaps as late as A.D. 429 (Blair, 1970). If rat populations had established themselves in the Roman townships then these towns would have had a nucleus of animals ready to expand as the town grew and became more populous. However, the continuation of the Roman urbanisation process was halted and settlements destroyed or left empty in the early part of the fifth century. If continuity is to be proved town life must be shown to have survived the sixth century and the evidence is that in only three centres – York, London and Canterbury – is there any suggestion of this by A.D. 597 and even then the claim to any status greater than that of village is tenuous (Hill, 1977). Loyn (1970) says:

> In contrast to the situation in Gaul the break in the continuity of town-life and villa-life was sharp and dramatic; even more clearly so with the villa than with the town. This is not to deny the possibility of continuity in habitation sites at places such as London, York or Cambridge ... Canterbury, although it changed its name from Durovernum, is one attested site for continuity, probably as a federal headquarters.

Continuity is also accepted for Dorchester.

There are 19 Anglo-Saxon towns on Roman sites but in only three of these is there any record of the setting up of a burh (defended centre). The three are

Colchester, Chester and Worcester. Ilchester was of no importance until the tenth century and in the cases of the remaining 15, archaeology has provided most of the evidence. In Winchester, where intensive excavation of the city began in 1960, it has been shown that there was a breakdown of urban life in the fifth century and there is reason for believing that there was only a thread of continuity to the early capital of the seventh century. Hill (1977) is also of the opinion that occupation, apart from the religious and royal centre, was on a small scale. Apart from the abbey, Gloucester had nothing to prove its importance before A.D. 850 and for Bath, Chichester and Dorchester there is no archaeological evidence. In the South-east, no Saxon levels have yet been found in Hastings and whilst trade passed through Dover in the mid-Saxon period it did not have any urban status. Both Cambridge and Lincoln have some early material but in neither case is it on such a scale that any major centres could be envisaged for the seventh century.

In addition to the three sites mentioned as showing some evidence of continuity must be added Rochester. The other sites are all re-foundations of the Age of Alfred and perhaps in two cases of Offa's Mercia. A few concentrations of pagan burials have been recorded near Canterbury and Cambridge and silver coins, *sceattas*, tell of considerable trade in the period A.D. 650–750 at a very few Roman towns that were *resettled*. As Hill (1977) points out, the correct word is resettled because no sixth-century population in these towns can be proved and all the impetus for starting afresh came from outside.

The Roman towns which were re-occupied owed their re-development to three major factors; their defensive nature, communications and the church. Communications were a decisive factor in choosing a site to settle and their importance and the topography of many Roman sites made it almost impossible for subsequent settlers to choose any other site if they wished to develop trade. For example, of 34 towns founded by the West Saxons between 840 and 925 (i.e. those 'burhs' which went on to become Domesday boroughs), 27 are associated with Roman roads, although ten sites were not Roman. St Albans was built afresh and the old road up Watling Street and through the site of Verulamium made a detour through the new town. The Roman occupation continued late at St Albans and the town may have been urban until the beginning of the sixth century but it has no mention in early records of Saxon history.

Because of this lack of urban continuity Rackham contends that the serious disease outbreaks recorded in the *Annals* were not likely to have been of bubonic plague which is essentially a disease of communities. These outbreaks occurred around the time that the epidemic of A.D. 542 was present in Europe. Morris (1973) considered this to be bubonic plague and talks of the great plague which devastated Ireland. Alcock (1971) quotes from the Welsh *Easter Annals* in which it was recorded that Maelgwn of Gwynedd died in 549 as a result of plague – *mortalitas magna*, the Great Plague. Both authors treat the epidemics in the *Annals* as part of the continental outbreak.

This question of the lack of continuity in urban life could be important in helping us to decide whether plague was present in Britain during Roman times and in the centuries following the departure of the Romans. Rackham has demonstrated the presence of *Rattus rattus* in a well in York and although the species may have been present in the highly organised towns and centrally heated villas of Roman Britain, the destruction of these towns appears to have been almost complete and this abrupt end would most likely have destroyed the rat populations since they would not have lasted long in the countryside without warm places in which to shelter. Rackham points out that if plague was present in Britain it would be expected to be severe in the towns of late Roman Britain with their extensive trade and constant travel. There is, however, no record either then or subsequently which leads us to think that the earlier widespread plagues, such as that in the time of Gallienus, were bubonic.

The vegetation cover, the type of agriculture and the sizes of settlements are features which must be considered in assessing the possibilities of the existence of rat populations in medieval England. Tansley (1968) pointed out that when he wrote, built-up areas made up about 10.6 per cent of the surface of England. Before World War II more than half of the whole area was grassland of one sort or another, less than a quarter was under arable crops, about one twentieth was woodland and more than one twentieth was heath, moorland and bog. The wartime ploughing campaign altered things so that whereas the percentage of tilled land in 1930 was 28 per cent, by 1944 it had increased to 48 per cent.

The vegetation at the time of the Roman occupation, i.e. in the later Iron Age, consisted of large areas of forest. Most of the English lowlands such as the Weald and the Midland Plain were largely covered with woodland which was mainly uninhabited while in the uplands of the west and north, oak forest covered the valley sides, giving way to pine and birch woods at higher altitudes and on the poorer, sandy soils. Ash was probably the main cover on the mountain limestones of North and South Pennines, perhaps covering the valley sides. The cultivated areas were found on the chalk and the loam soils of the South-east.

The Romans destroyed much forest but agriculture was probably increased during the occupation and there was probably little effect on the vegetation as a whole. The occupation changed the rural economy but little for most Roman activities were concerned with building towns and roads. The great forests remained in the South, on the Weald, in South-west Essex and the Midland Plain and woodland was extensive between the villages of the native population and the Roman villa farms. Except for hunting, the larger forests were probably little traversed. The iron sands on the Weald led to smelting and the use of trees for providing charcoal must have made some inroads into the forest.

The coming of the Saxons in the fifth century A.D. saw the cultivation of the lowlands begin and the clearing of forests from valleys and low-lying plains, but woodland was still very extensive. The Saxons at first occupied the lighter loam soils of the South-east. The Celts were driven into the west and thus the cultivation of the chalk uplands almost ceased. Even if rats had survived the destruction of Roman towns, a species as dependent upon man as *R. rattus* would have been in a precarious position and only in a few seaports could animals have survived.

In order to subjugate the Saxons the Normans destroyed large portions of many counties, burned crops and houses and killed farm animals. Land so badly used probably reverted to the wild state for some years. The kings formed the 'Royal Forests' for hunting and forbade most cultivation within them. These forests consisted of heath and moorland as well as trees and it is said that they covered one-third of the country by the mid twelfth century.[9] At this stage the afforestation policy was reversed and from now on the extension of pasturage and agriculture carried on through the Middle Ages. As forest was cleared for tilling, the grazing of cattle and pigs in the forest went on, the cattle being responsible for destruction of forest and the swine assisting in regeneration.

Platt (1978) points out that in relation to its natural resources and the quality of its technology, England was seriously overpopulated at the beginning of the fourteenth century. The desire for land by the peasants had pushed arable farming into less suitable soils and broken down the existing land units into fragments which were less viable on their own. As the population rose and pasture receded before arable, the village livestock declined in number. This saw the beginning of a vicious circle of events: the loss of pasture pushed up the price beyond reach of the poor and the lack of meat led to protein deficiencies in poor villagers. The lack of manure caused the already low levels of productivity to fall further with soil exhaustion probably severe on smaller holdings.

This overpopulation has been the subject of much comment by historians. Titow (1961–2) showed that the thirteenth century was a period of population growth. Between 1209 and 1311 the male population of the Somerset manor of Taunton rose from 612 to 1448. This was equivalent to a cumulative annual rate of increase of 0.85 per cent and was almost twice the rate of the population increase in England over the eighteenth century (0.44 per cent) although below the modern Indian figure of 1.3 per cent. Titow considered that the Winchester Account Rolls provide good indications that the famines of 1315, 1316 and 1317 marked the turning point in this upward trend for the number of persons paying the hundred penny payment (this was a payment of a penny from every male person over 12 years of age) dropped considerably after these famines.

Harvey (1966) concluded that much of English society was living at the Malthusian level of subsistence by 1300 and that during the next 20 or 25 years the trend of the previous two centuries or more was reversed. Various other studies have all reached some agreement that the English population had reached a peak by or during the early part of the fourteenth century, e.g. Russell (1966), Hallam (1961–2), the latter author showing that in 1300 the Lincolnshire fenland had a population comparable in size with that of the mid-twentieth century.

Throughout the Middle Ages arable cultivation extended in the form of open fields cultivated in common and belonging to the village communities. Forests were still extensive and important: people had pasture rights and were allowed to collect dead wood, almost their sole source of fuel. Due to grazing, forests must have degraded into poor grassland or heath on which grew bushes resistant to grazing. In the Middle Ages farming for profit replaced subsistence farming and the proportions of arable and pasture fluctuated with the prices of corn and wool and cloth. Textiles became a major medieval industry and sheep achieved great prominence.

It follows from this that the population was not evenly distributed over rural Britain. If it had been uniform throughout England and Wales the resulting density would have been 63 per square mile but, if spread evenly over England alone, 69 per square mile. Shrewsbury has made some calculations from Russell (1948) on the population density of counties per square mile but, using the conversion factor suggested by Russell to arrive at a 1346 figure, I cannot find very close agreement with Shrewsbury and in fact his figure of the population density of England and Wales was 69 per square mile. These differences probably mean little but, taking the five most densely populated counties (Table 3), it can be seen that my calculated densities are lower than those given by Shrewsbury. The positions of Northamptonshire and Suffolk are reversed and Rutland occupies the fifth position with Leicestershire moving down. The five least densely populated counties are more affected with Cheshire moving from top to bottom position. Of this second group Shewsbury says that these densities, i.e. between 20 and 25 per square mile on his calculations but 19 to 32 on mine, are so low that it would have been *biologically impossible* for bubonic plague to have spread over any of these counties in the fourteenth century, though it might by chance have been introduced into one or more of their towns and villages. Unfortunately, we have too little objective information from plague epidemics this century to provide us with any indication of the minimum human population density necessary to sustain an epidemic. In fact it is probably impossible to arrive at such a figure because of habitat differences. For example, plague might be widely evident in tropical Vietnam where the continuous dense vegetation provided conditions suitable for epizootics in widespread rat populations whilst in Arabia, at the same human density per square mile, the vast expanse of desert would ensure that rats only existed in townships.

Despite what Shrewsbury says about the biological impossibility of plague at these densities that disease, or something else, was present and fairly

TABLE 3

Population densities (persons/square mile) in English counties in 1346

(Data calculated from Russell, 1948)

Highest density counties (Shrewsbury calculation)		Lowest density counties (Shrewsbury calculation)		Middle density counties (Twigg calculation)
County	*Density*	*County*	*Density*	*96–81 per sq. mile*
Norfolk	119	Cheshire	25	Buckinghamshire; Leicestershire;
Bedfordshire		Westmorland		Oxfordshire; Cambridgeshire;
Suffolk	➔	Durham	➔	Middlesex; Hertfordshire;
Northamptonshire		Northumberland		Huntingdonshire; Kent;
Leicestershire	101	Cumberland	20	Lincolnshire; Nottinghamshire.
				80–71 per sq. mile
(Twigg calculation)		(Twigg calculation)		Dorset; Essex; Gloucestershire;
				Somerset; Warwickshire.
Norfolk	109	Westmorland	32	
Bedfordshire	105	Northumberland	29	*70–61 per sq. mile*
Northamptonshire	100	Cumberland	28	Berkshire; Cornwall; Yorkshire.
Suffolk	99	Durham	24	
Rutland	98	Cheshire	19	*60–33 per sq. mile*
				Devon; Derbyshire; Hampshire;
				Herefordshire; Lancashire;
				Shropshire; Staffordshire;
				Surrey; Sussex; Worcestershire.

widespread in Cheshire to judge from the map in Shrewsbury where the maximum possible percentage mortality among beneficed clergy ranged from 20 in the Nantwich deanery to 66 in Middlewich. In the four northern counties the epidemic was recorded in Durham and perhaps from New-castle-upon-Tyne in Northumberland. There are no records of the disease from the diocese of Carlisle (this consisted of most of the parishes in Cumberland, together with those in the northern half of Westmorland) because there are no records for the period in question. The scarcity of records is a major problem generally and especially unfortunate for such a large area as this.

Between the two extremes the densities range from 96 to 33 per square mile (Table 3). Shrewsbury says that the epidemiology of bubonic plague makes it improbable that *Y. pestis* could have been distributed by rat-contacts as epizootic plague in any English county in 1348–9 having an average population density of less than 60 per square mile. Nevertheless, the disease, whatever it was, appears to have been extensive in ten counties having less than 60 persons per square mile (apart from the five already mentioned which had 19 to 32 per square mile). These ten counties were Devon, Derbyshire, Hampshire, Herefordshire, Lancashire, Shropshire, Staffordshire, Surrey, Sussex and Worcestershire. Given the uneven spread of communities within the counties, e.g. Derbyshire, the expression of density on a county basis is probably of limited value.

Of his figure of 69 per square mile Shrewsbury says that if we allow an average of five persons per dwelling[10] and ignore the aggregation of people in towns, villages, castles and monasteries, there would not have been more than 14 dwellings to the square mile in Britain for the house-rat to infest. Even if one supposes that there was an average of *100 rats* (my italics) in each dwelling, which he agrees is almost certainly an excessive allowance for the two-room cottages which constituted most of the dwellings, then the density of the overall house-rat population would have been too low to engender and sustain an epizootic of rat-plague on a national scale. He calculates that if all the 14 dwellings had been grouped in compact hamlets the local concent-rations of house-rats might have been able to support localised epizootics, with consequent local plague epidemics among the villagers but the long distances which separated the hamlets would have minimised the risk of either kind of plague becoming widespread. Shrewsbury considers that if the manorial and monastic groupings are included there must have been many large areas of land in which there were neither sufficient human beings nor house-rats to provide subjects for *Y. pestis*, and these empty spaces must have acted as effective barriers to the spread of the disease.

He concludes his observations on this question with the comment that only the towns in fourteenth-century England provided sufficiently large aggregations of house-rats for dangerous epizootics of rat-plague to develop, and points out that there were few towns with populations exceeding 5,000 persons. London, the largest town, had a population of around 58,000 and only four other towns exceeded 10,000. These were Bristol (c. 15,800), Coventry (c. 12,000), Plymouth (c. 12,000) and York (c. 18,000) with Norwich close behind at c. 9,800.

Shrewsbury considered that most of the fourteenth-century towns were separated by areas in which the concentrations of house-rats were so low that plague could not have spread from one to another along rat pipelines as he called them (i.e. a continuous rat to rat contact) but could only have occurred as a result of the chance transport of infected rats or blocked fleas. Pointing out the large areas of uninhabited forest, waste and fenland he observes that with the exception of a few hamlets on their margins, the moorlands of Yorkshire, Somerset, Devon and Wales were devoid of human and rat life. They probably were but it is difficult to be entirely sure about this.

An important point in Shrewsbury's argument about plague spread was the grouping of most habitations into villages with very few outlying farms. He was of the opinion that farms would have served as links in the transmission of plague from one village and its population of rats to the next. But, even if such farms had existed and had had rats it is difficult to see how this would have provided the link because in the climate of the British Isles *Rattus rattus* does not leave buildings and would not therefore have provided a rat pipeline. Finally, Shrewsbury concludes that from what is now known of the aetiology of bubonic plague it was therefore a '*biological impossibility for the whole or even a major part of England to have been ravaged by "The Great Pestilence" of 1348–50*'.

This is a most important statement when one looks at the volume of data in Shrewsbury and elsewhere which shows that a large part of Britain, rural as well as urban, was affected at the time under consideration. If there was this difficulty about rats being present, which Shrewsbury sees, then he is correct in saying that it was impossible for 'The Great Pestilence' to have had this effect, providing he means, as he mainly does, that 'The Great Pestilence' was bubonic plague. If there was this lack of rats the whole case for bubonic plague is less certain. If, though, another disease, not rat-borne, was the major factor in the pestilence then the absence of rats is no barrier to spread in either town or countryside.

Shrewsbury clearly appreciated the limitations imposed by climate upon *Rattus rattus* for he says that although it is cautious, it does not avoid man and in temperate latitudes like Britain it can only survive with the aid of the shelter provided by human habitation. Yet he has to imply the outdoor presence of rats, even in autumn, when referring to plague spread in Dorset he talks about a creeping epizootic, which implies continuous rat populations across the countryside. Hamlets and villages – the only rural dwellings – were so scattered that even if they harboured rats there could be no contact between the separate rat groups. Shrewsbury says that at the present time the chief habitats of *Rattus rattus* outside its Indian home appear to be the seaports of

99

both tropical and temperate lands. This is not strictly true, but it is likely that it was always so in Britain where it was also found in those inland towns connected to the ports by canals (Bentley, 1959). The Black rat is much more widespread in the tropics than Shrewsbury indicates for it is in some places the common rat of the countryside.

An important aspect of plague spread is the continuity across a rat population. The more isolated the rat units the slower will be the movement of plague amongst rats and, ultimately, to people. In the warmer parts of the world *Rattus rattus* is found away from buildings but in Britain, because of the climate, it is an indoor animal. In ports where there exist blocks of multi-storied buildings, this handicap does not hinder its fairly rapid spread but districts consisting of streets of semi-detached houses, no matter how many carelessly maintained dust-bins and chicken runs are present, are a barrier to it, as are open spaces and wide thoroughfares. In order to cross these it must be transported by man (Bentley, 1959). Even the Brown rat, which has less temperature constraints, is loth to cross city streets and rat populations in grid plan North American cities live out their lives within the same block.

An examination of the plans of some Anglo-Saxon towns reveals that in many cases a surprisingly rectangular pattern of blocks of buildings was evident. Winchester shows a clear grid plan: the city's overall dimensions being about 750 m × 600 m, with city blocks at maximum 110 m wide and 20 m at the minimum. Late-Saxon Winchester, c. A.D. 993–1066, had grown to 800 m × 650 m, still on a rectangular grid plan, with twelve rectangular blocks approximately 280 m × 100 m, and Hereford in the Saxon period, c. A.D. 700–1066, was roughly 600 m × 600 m (Biddle, 1976).

Many planted towns after 1066 were based on the grid. Beresford (1967) lists 26 English towns which exhibit surviving clear grid plans. Amongst these are Melcombe Regis, founded by 1268, Portsmouth by 1194, Liverpool by 1207, King's Lynn 1086–95 and Stratford upon Avon by 1196. A further 26 Welsh towns show the same plan, including Carnarvon, Monmouth, Conway and Beaumaris, all founded during the same period. Thus, by the arrival of the Great Pestilence there was much evidence of grid planning in the towns. Another town plan was that based on the market, seen in such towns as Devizes, Pembroke and Newton Abbot (Butler, 1976). In this plan, plots were concentrated around the market place and with no other streets to divide the plots there were, therefore, no chequers. A third plan was the ribbon based plan. By the seventeenth century towns covered a considerable area. Hereford, for example, was 750 m × 700 m; Ely 1000 m × 600 m and Chester the same (Platt, 1976).

Tout (1917) in an essay on medieval town planning says that the rectilinear alignment and rectangular blocks of allotments have been common to town planners of every age and points to the older parts of the older cities of Prussia, Silesia, Poland and Lithuania as showing this pattern, a particularly good example being the regular gridding of Breslau.

The generally held impression of fourteenth-century towns being a jumble of buildings, contiguous one with another across the length and breadth of the town, is seen to be erroneous in fact. The Black rat, if present, would probably have been as strictly confined to blocks in the Winchester of 1348 as it is in the San Francisco of the twentieth century and, because of the lower temperature, would have been perhaps even more restricted. The spread of plague across a city would have been a slow event and the account of it going through Genoa in a couple of days, if accurate, could under no circumstances refer to plague.

Most of the population of Britain lived in the countryside in settlements which were usually small villages and we know that there were many of these. Although all had certain features in common, the shape of the village was dictated by the type of husbandry carried out or the industry on which the village was supported. Some villages were strung out along a road; these obtained their livelihood from the traffic which passed along the road. Villages whose industry was based on cloth tended to contain more smallholdings or cottages closely packed together than was usual whilst coal, iron and tin-mining villages as well as fishing settlements tended to be spread out.

A large proportion of the rural population lived by agriculture. The large areas of monoculture which today so favour pests either at the growing stage or in the storage of large amounts of food did not exist then. The arable land was divided into strips, each often less than one acre, and different peoples' land would be intermingled in a seemingly extraordinary confusion although the rules governing distribution of land and the crops grown were very carefully ordered. Slater (1907) has reviewed the various types of village agricultural systems on a regional basis and shown how the enclosures of common fields altered the agricultural system and the countryside to a marked degree.

The main feature of the village was that it was a grouped settlement and the shape most commonly seen was the 'nucleated' village in which the houses were tightly clustered round some feature which made a natural centre for the group such as the church or the village green (Postan, 1975). Each cottage had a small plot of land behind it for growing vegetables (Neilson, 1941), the arable land lay around the village and beyond this extended the 'waste' and forests.

Each manor may have had a mill. Although there was a great deal of self-sufficiency this has been exaggerated. According to Coulton (1949) there would be coming and going on the busier roads but these were comparatively rare. Outside, the ways or tracks were not designed for continuous travel; they made only for the nearest village and the nearest market might well be too distant to be worth while. Apart from occasional pedlars, wandering friars and travelling artisans the average medieval villager was probably more cut off from the world than we can envisage today (Coulton, 1949). Postan (1975) gives an admirable account of the medieval economy and society.

Bennett (1938) described the peasant house typical of those found North and West of a line from the Wash to the Bristol Channel. These were 'cruck' houses, the crucks being the main timbers, curved uprights placed opposite each other and forming a fork in which a ridge-pole fitted. The ridge-pole ran the length of the house and held the various pairs of uprights firmly together. The roof ran from the ridge-pole to the ground and the space within the house was severely limited. When Britain was extensively forested it must have been fairly easy to find a tree naturally bent in such a form that it was easily adapted to form a fork. The type of structure with curved uprights gave more room than this in the lower part of the house. From this developed a later house style with the lower portion constructed of heavy timbers forming the corners and intermediate posts and standing eight or ten feet up from the foundations, thus giving more room than the curved upright form.

There were few instances of stone walls, even in good stone country. Almost everywhere wattle and daub (or cob), with turf and mud were the main materials (Clifton-Taylor, 1972; Muir, 1980). Wattle and daub consisted of a number of sticks stuck upright, with twigs woven in and out to form a sort of lattice onto which was thrown the *dab* until it was of the right thickness. Such buildings probably burned well and they may have soon deteriorated. Beresford and Hurst (1979) were of the opinion that peasant houses of the time were probably rebuilt about every generation, the frequent rebuilding suggesting that the roofs were not properly carpentered but were simple structures of undressed timber and branches. Most cottages were thatched, always with a straw of some kind. In Lincolnshire and Norfolk, reeds were abundant and made good roofs. In some areas bracken was the main material. It has been suggested that such buildings were very fragile. For example, it is said that thieves could break in with ease through walls or doors and there is a record of a man being killed at his own fireside by a spear thrust in through the house wall. Windows were few and small since glass was too expensive for the peasant who covered the small window opening with a wooden shutter which excluded both light and air (cf. India). There were no chimneys, only a louvre in the roof to let out the smoke (Neilson, 1941).

Such dwellings were small (Rowley, 1978). The specification of one which a new tenant is bound to build to house a predecessor is as follows: 'He is to build her a competent dwelling for her to inhabit, containing 30 feet in length within the walls, and 14 feet in breadth, with corner posts and three new and competent doors and two windows' (Coulton, 1925). A specification of 1325 describes a cottage 24 feet × 11 feet to house a man and his wife and son.

In a small cottage like this the roof would be the only secure place for rats to live and in the British climate, unable to forage outside, they would be either easily detected and destroyed or would be unlikely to contact other rats in neighbouring houses. It is difficult to see large numbers building up under these conditions.

A point to bear in mind about rats in general and *Rattus rattus* in particular is that they thrive under conditions of food storage, especially when this is on a large scale and there is less fear of detection and disturbance. It was a feature of medieval populations that they did not store food to any degree and this was one reason why a harvest failure was such a catastrophe. There was, therefore, little chance of this feature aiding population build-up either.

On the continent of Europe the housing was much the same. M. Simeon Luce studied the period and described the structure of huts in rural France in 1348 (in Gasquet, 1908). There was very seldom any masonry. They were mostly merely four mud, or clay, walls, sometimes wickerwork lined with the interstices filled in with hay and straw. They were single-storied with a roof which was thatched or covered with wood or stone.

Older in origin than the cruck cottage is the long-house, found all over Europe among pastoral folk in wild, mountainous regions. This consists of a long, low rectangular building housing family and cattle under one roof. Patterns vary from region to region but usually the living room adjoined the cow house with direct access and no more divisions than a partitioned feeding walk. There was usually a central hearth and a loft above. Edwards (1972) and Peate (1944) give detailed accounts of cruck and long-houses. Figure 7 shows a plan of a typical long-house from Gwndwn, Pencader, Carmarthenshire (after Peate, 1944). Clearly, such a building with its overhead loft and cow feed, plenty of cover and darkness would have been much more suitable for rat harbourage but their situation is mainly in the regions which would be least hospitable to the Black rat.

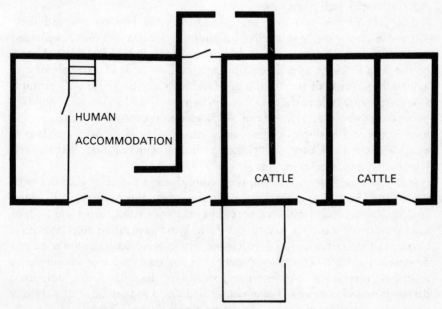

Fig. 7 A long-house from Carmarthenshire.

Harvey (1965) gives a detailed description of the Oxfordshire village of Cuxham between 1240 and 1400 and includes some details of construction. About 1315 in the manor house the lord's room with the latrine, which was probably adjoining, was the only building roofed with shingles. It was built of stone and reached by wooden steps and had several unglazed windows. These must have ensured a cold building, despite the presence of shutters. The hall was a wooden-framed building with walls of wattle and daub. Both it and all the remaining domestic buildings had tiled roofs, with the exception of a room next to the kitchen which was thatched.

All the farm buildings which were newly built or extensively reconstructed between 1310 and 1330 were given tiled roofs. Earlier, all but the granary and the dovecotes had been thatched, so the use of tiles had extended beyond the domestic buildings of the manor house (although these buildings still belonged to the manor farm and it is very unlikely that tiled roofs were ever found on peasant dwellings). The new roofing style did not extend all over because the lease of the manor in 1420 refers to both tiled and thatched buildings, as exists today.

From the late twelfth century the merchants of Southamton (Platt, 1973) lived in good stone houses and at the same time merchant houses made entirely of stone, roofed with tile and slate began to appear in Lincoln, Norwich, Bury St Edmunds and Canterbury (Platt, 1978). Although fashion had some part to play in the change from thatch to roofs of tiles and slate, the need for fire-proofing was evident since some of these houses by the fourteenth century possessed good quality tiled floors, painted window glass and sometimes wall paintings.

The fear of fire was ever present. During the late twelfth and early thirteenth centuries the municipal building regulations of London provided against fire and in large houses the kitchens were built detached through most of the Middle Ages as a precaution against fire. A good example of this approach was that of the Bishop of Hereford's manor house at Prestbury, Gloucestershire, where the detached kitchen was linked to the main building by a pentice about 20 metres long. Archaeological excavations of the period have uncovered examples of fires to isolated buildings (Wilson and Hurst, 1964; Webster and Cherry, 1975) and to whole streets and areas (Webster and Cherry, 1974; Carter et al., 1977).

It is interesting to compare peasant conditions in medieval England with those found in the Indian peasant community early this century. In Belgaum (Plague Research Commission, 1910) houses were single-storied and built of mud with outer walls one to two feet thick. Most were raised on plinths built of mud but in most cases faced with stone. Floors were made of mud or beaten down earth with a layer of cow dung and the roofs were of country tiles resting on several layers of interlacing bamboos, the whole being supported by rough wooden beams. These houses had up to four rooms but only one door to the outside, windows, if present, being boarded up.

Every house had a store of grain, usually kept in sacks in the living room but occasionally in cylindrical receptacles made of bamboo matting. Many houses had a platform inside them, six or seven feet high, made of bamboos and supported on bamboo uprights, which served as a store for fodder, stores and rubbish.

Cattle often shared houses with the people and the Commission recorded that the overcrowding was appalling. The worst instance seen was in a house of three fairly large rooms and a verandah which was occupied by the following: 12 adults; three children; four buffaloes; six bullocks; one goat; one dog; one cat and three fowls. Whilst this was an extreme case, conditions nearly as bad were not uncommon. In the houses of the poor and lower middle class, beds were rarely seen in Belgaum although they were common in the Punjab. We have no such figures on house sharing with domestic animals in Britain and although the long-house is the nearest equivalent, even there the cattle were some distance away from people.

The Indian survey of a plague area provides some illuminating facts on rat presence and animals. In Belgaum city, excluding the suburbs, there were 23,885 people in 3,813 inhabited dwelling houses, i.e. 6.3 people per house and in Sadar Bazaar 5.5 people per house. In both areas there were many uninhabited houses but, since most of these were shops, godowns and stores, they may have been very important in harbouring and feeding rats. In 14 months in the city 8.6 rats per house were caught – that is one rat every 1.6 months. During 12 months in Sadar Bazaar 8.3 rats per house were caught. It is interesting to compare some more recent estimates of rat populations in modern cities. Davis (1950) estimated that the Brown rat population of New York in 1949 was not more than 250,000 or one rat for 36 persons, and in Baltimore in 1949 (Davis and Fales, 1950) to be about 60,000 or one rat per 15 inhabitants. The comparisons are not easy to make with Belgaum because the Indian figures refer to rats caught whilst the American ones are estimates of total rat numbers.

In Belgaum the harbouring of domestic animals in houses increased the number of rats caught but not by very much. Those houses which had one or more of buffaloes, bullocks, cows, ponies or goats per house averaged 9.2 rats per house and houses with no domestic animals had 8.3 rats. Roughly similar figures were found in Sadar Bazaar – 9.6 rats in houses with domestic animals and 8.2 in those without. Thus the keeping of animals in the house only slightly favoured rat infestation, the extra food supply not having a marked influence.

Some buildings in Belgaum had heavy infestations, one grocer's shop having more than 100 rats caught in the year. Another house of three rooms had six people *and two cats* yet 197 rats were caught in the year. Of 17 houses in which more than 50 but less than 100 rats were caught, nine were dwelling houses, two were grocers, one was a grain godown, two were liquor shops, one was a butcher's shop, one a stable and one a weaver's house. Of 237 houses having more than 20 but less than 50 rats, 24 were grocers, sweet-meat sellers or grain stores and 27 were weavers or tailors.

Plague was more severe in the Bazaar than in the city, due, it was said, to the greater rat populations although the figures given show only a small increase in rat numbers. The Bazaar had a higher proportion of cats than the city; one to every 124 people as against one to 760, but this was apparently not enough to eradicate the rats.

As a further comparison with possible conditions in medieval England the features and rat infestations of Egyptian houses in 1912 when plague was active can be cited (Petrie and Todd, 1923). An epidemic of plague occurred in Qûs Town in January to April 1912 and the investigators examined a typical plague house, showing how the structural features were related to rat infestation and rat plague. The building was a typical dwelling house in Upper Egypt, made of burnt bricks with an upper floor and flat roof; it enclosed three sides of a courtyard, which was bounded on the remaining side by the wall of an adjacent house. Five rooms opened into the courtyard from the ground floor, one of them being used as a store-room for fodder and another as a stable for donkeys and domestic animals. The courtyard served as an animal-yard and fowl-run; a heap of rubbish and building debris occupied much of it.

The living rooms on the upper floor were reached by a brick staircase and were entered from balconies built over the courtyard. On the flat roof were two small rooms. The floors of the upper rooms and balconies consisted of a double layer of burnt bricks bound together with clay; they were supported by the lath-like stems of palm-tree leaves which were laid across stout beams made of split palm-tree trunks. The ground-floor rooms had a ceiling formed by sheets of matting, rotted away in some places.

During their first visit the investigators noted the distinctive smell of decomposing rats and found a sick *R. rattus* crouching near a courtyard wall. This animal was later shown to be plague-infected. In this house the focus of infection was the shaft of the cesspit which led from a privy on the floor above to the pit below. A narrow passage around the shaft led to the courtyard by means of an inadequately bricked arch and from the floor of the passage 30 dead rats were removed. A dead infected rat lay near the privy opening and rat burrows tracked into and around the cesspit shaft. By clearing the bricks round the privy the burrows were partly exposed and six dead rats were found.

A technique employed by plague investigators for finding plague-infected fleas in premises was to run flea-free guinea-pigs which would attract rat fleas whose hosts had died. In this case a guinea-pig left to run in the space at the base of the cesspit shaft for three days collected 684 rat fleas and died of plague. Fleas taken from this animal were put on a healthy guinea-pig which also died of plague.

When the infectivity of the house was judged to have ended the cesspit shaft was demolished for examination. 53 dead rats and one *Acomys*, a local rodent, were found. Examination of the house structure revealed that the clay between bricks had become pulverised so as to form spaces which contained many dead rats and in addition dead rats were picked up from the floors of most rooms.

After disinfection a guinea-pig was placed in each of eight rooms: five of them died of plague. In view of the structure it is presumed that many more dead rats, and fleas, were present in the fabric but this could only have been determined by taking the house apart. Nevertheless, the severity of the infection was obvious and was in all probability characteristic of many such dwellings. Clearly, both rats and fleas were abundant and in close contact with the human inhabitants. In the survey of plague in Egypt, between 90 and 100 per cent of *X. cheopis* found on *Rattus rattus*, *Rattus norvegicus*, *Acomys cahirinus* and *Arvicanthis niloticus* were from houses. The following shows the number of fleas and the range per rat:

Rodent	Flea numbers (range/species of rodent)
Rattus rattus	1.7–11.1
Acomys cahirinus	0.2–0.83
Rattus norvegicus	1.3–32.6

These were large numbers, especially on the two rat species and will be referred to again in Chapter 9 when I examine recent plague in Britain.

In the light of this plague reservoir it might have been expected that there would have been a massive plague outbreak. The town of Qûs contained 15,000 people with some degree of crowding, a climate favourable to flea breeding and many rats of both plague-carrying species yet there were only 82 cases. Of these, 51 were bubonic, 16 had no obvious buboes and 15 were pneumonic. In view of the latter cases there was scope for rapid spread of the disease and I shall return to this point again, as well as to the next feature, the timing of the sick cases. The first case occurred on 14 January, the next on 26 February, five of this household being taken ill later, and between 26 February and 9 March there were ten more cases, but no more cases there until the middle of April. Thus, there were only 17 cases in the first 13 weeks of the outbreak, a state of affairs oddly at variance with most medieval accounts. There were 61 deaths, 74 per cent of the cases, and whilst this was a high case mortality (but quite usual before antibiotics) it seems nevertheless to have been a remarkably small number of plague victims.

Plague in the third pandemic in Egypt provided field evidence on an outbreak of the disease in small villages, similar in size to those of medieval England and with perhaps many other features in common, including poverty and a primitive way of life. The Kôm Ombo agricultural estate, situated on the bank of the Nile 520 miles (836 km) south of Cairo and 30 miles (48 km) north of Aswan, comprised about 23,000 acres with 29 hamlets in which an average of 250 persons dwelt. The total population was 12,831 in 1912. However, the estate was of recent origin, about ten years old, and was a centre for casual labour. On account of its recency the settlers did not constitute a fixed population.

Plague first appeared in January 1911 in several hamlets and many workers fled in panic to their native districts. Some of these people already had plague and were traced later. There were 357 cases of plague with 237 deaths (66.4 per cent) from January to the end of April but this figure was thought to be an underestimate. Even so it was very low compared with medieval outbreaks. In two hamlets, one with a population of 920 had eight cases of bubonic and septicaemic plague and the other with 364 people had 20 cases. The latter village was less than one year old and had about 100 mud houses, some in rows back-to-back and others in single rows. The houses were very simple: each consisted of a single room six feet square, with mud floor and walls and with a straw roof supported by a pole. The mud walls were thicker at ground level than at the top. Many owners had added a small courtyard in which to stable the larger domestic animals.

Extraordinarily high rat-flea numbers were taken from individual houses, e.g. 15, 120, 1005, 3051 and 430. On taking one house apart a system of rat nests and burrows was found which clearly communicated with adjacent houses. Mummified *R. norvegicus* and *Arvicanthis niloticus* were found in the nests and burrows.

Finally, a third epidemic in Abnûb town between January and April 1912 produced 48 bubonic or septicaemic cases in a population of 16,000 people, again a low incidence compared with epidemics of the Middle Ages.

Compared with Belgaum the rodent population per house in Upper Egypt was low and averaged out at, for example in El Motiâ, 1.22 *R. rattus* and 1.24 *Acomys* per dwelling although individual houses may have had as many as 19 *R. rattus* and four *Acomys*. Each house had, on average, 14 rat holes in its fabric.

As in India, the houses served the double function of dwelling place and animal stable, a combination then seen often in Upper Egypt. Goats, donkeys, sheep and fowls shared with the owners and camels, oxen and buffaloes were tethered in enclosures annexed to each house. It had been expected that the stone houses would be less rodent infested than the mud houses but this was not so because the stone dwellings were structurally defective, the foundations being built of unsquared, indifferently cemented stones. Grain pits proved to be focal points for rat fleas and, presumably, rats too, the flea data for two such pits being seen in Table 4.

Conditions in medieval England cannot be analysed so precisely because of our lack of knowledge. Shrewsbury maintains that the reason why bubonic plague was chiefly a disease of the poor was because of the nature of the roofing material in homes below the rank of manor. These people, he said,

TABLE 4

Flea counts on guinea-pigs isolated in grain-pits in a stone house at Atmour Bahari, Egypt

Flea counts on successive days

| | Day | | | | | | | | | | Total number of fleas |
	1	2	3	4	5	6	7	8	9	10	
Pit A	1064	599	510	303	265	356	242	136	365	246	4,086
Pit B	324	280	136	97	150	69	90	43	289	70	1,548

TOTAL: 5,634

Pit A: Deep grain-pit 1.5 × 1.0 m: 1.25 m deep.
Pit B: Shallow grain-pit 1.0 × 1.0 m: 60 cm deep.

lived in single-storey huts, roofed with thatch or turf in which rats lived, bred and died and from whose nests starving 'blocked' fleas fell on the human occupants. Conversely, he reasons that the castles and manor houses with stone or wooden walls and stone roofs would give no shelter to the house-rat since all had at least one storey and many had two or three above the ground floor and thus the occupants would be exempt from rat-flea attack. But the Black rat is a good climber and it could surely have found harbourage between floors. There would also be more food in a castle, more grain stored and, because of the greater affluence, more waste. In a peasant hovel the poor would very likely consume every scrap of food.

Sanitation of the home must be considered as a factor encouraging rats. It is unlikely that human excreta provides food for rats except when they are starving, but the provision of a dark cesspit shaft which rats might inhabit and from which they might pass into various floors of a building could be important as we have seen in Egypt. In Belgaum (Plague Research Commission, 1910) most houses had latrines which were cleaned at night by city sweepers. In other places in India many houses had cesspits and these were rarely cleaned.

There is no information on the role of the privy in English peasant life and it seems likely that it was most probably an earth closet removed some distance from the cottage and still found in remote rural areas today. In monasteries and the ancient establishments of the wealthy, landed nobility, garderobes were part of the structure. Sometimes, as at Langley Castle, Northumberland, one of the principal towers would be used for this, with four separate garderobes built for each storey and with separate flues for filth from each passing down through the stonework of the tower to a stream at the bottom. Smaller turrets were sometimes used and when there was running water in the moat some of this was diverted through the pit of the garderobe.

We know something about sanitation in medieval London through the work of Sabine (1934). It seems that, whenever possible, privies were built in chambers corbelled out over the water of a moat or on arches over the water, with pipe drains to moats or with cesspools to receive the excreta. The latter method was employed when there was no running water. In 1259–60 a great innovation was tried when an underground sewer was built to carry away the filth from the royal kitchens and such drains or sewers to serve the garderobes of the palace were built around this time or soon afterwards.

As early as 1290–91 and 1312–13 public latrines existed for householders who had no private latrines and as late as 1579 in the parish of All Hallows, 57 households containing 85 people had only three privies. This state of affairs led to insanitary practices and in Basinghall Ward in 1421 all the little rents of the Swan were without privies and all the tenants threw ordures and waste before their doors. Nevertheless, not everyone favoured this and in 1307 there was an incident showing that public opinion was in favour of making wayfarers use public conveniences instead of relieving themselves in the streets. There were at least 13 public latrines in London and probably many more. The one on London Bridge was large, with several 'necessary houses'; in 1358 there were 138 shops on the Bridge and therefore a considerable need for adequate latrines. They were usually over water and private latrines were also built over water, a practice which became common until about 1462–3. There were also some sewerage systems for better-off citizens, like the one in Westminster Palace where the excreta passed from latrines via latrine pipes to cesspits.

If rats existed in fourteenth-century London, one aspect of life which would have sustained populations would have been the butchering practices. Cattle were butchered in the city, the blood flowing into the streets, and butchers threw remnants, scraps and dung into the highway. The pestilence was instrumental in causing agitation against butchers' filth: for example in the half century 1300–50 there were only two entries in the records on the agitation concerning butchers' filth, whereas in the period 1350–1400 there were 21 (Sabine, 1933).

Each outbreak of disease in the fourteenth century caused an outcry against the infection caused by butchers' filth. It would be interesting to know whether animal flesh was in some way held responsible for the epidemics. In the time of Queen Elizabeth I the slaughtering of animals within the city was looked upon as the cause of an outbreak of plague.

In 1301–2 certain butchers were charged with throwing animal remains into the King's highway and were told to carry such waste to the river and throw it in at the ebb-tide. Eventually, butchers were allowed to build a pier over the Thames with houses on it where they could cast offal into the river at ebb-tide, but it had first to be cut into small pieces.

Most towns were probably similar in these difficulties. Cambridge was so insanitary that when Henry III granted a charter to the town in 1267 one of the provisions was that it should be cleaned and the water-course opened (Williamson, 1957). This was not done and in 1388, in preparation for a meeting of Parliament in Cambridge, the King (Richard II) sent a writ to the Chancellor of the University requiring him to see that the town was cleaned up. Despite the Act of 1388, the troubles persisted and the streets and rivers were persistently fouled with garbage and intestines of slain beasts, carcasses and other filth. In Cambridge it was not apparently permitted to make a privy over the common river and the King's ditch and in 1502 the master of Buckingham College, the master or keeper of Clement Hostel and the keeper of Trinity Hall were all charged with this misdemeanour.

City cleaning, or the endeavours to get the populace to be more clean in their habits, was an uphill task. London, by virtue of its site on the north bank of the Thames and its close relationship with the Fleet Stream and Walbrook, which flowed through the centre of the city, used both these tributaries of the Thames in cleaning filth from the city. The wider streets had one gutter each side and the narrow ones had one down the centre. These had a water flow resulting from rainwater, well water and slops. In medieval times there was a highly organised system to take care of cleaning the city, from aldermen controlling each ward down to 'surveyors of pavement', four to each ward (Sabine, 1937) and city rakers who carted the muck away. As early as 1357 they had horses and carts for this purpose. Once again the epidemics of the second half of the fourteenth century focused attention on cleaning and there was a marked improvement in the sanitation conditions after the inauguration of stricter regulations. The entries in the Letter Books requiring action over cleaning were more numerous in the 50 years from 1350–1400 (65) than in the other 150 years of the 200 years from 1300–1500 (49) (Sabine, 1937).

One very curious fact emerges from a large number of records of complaints about refuse, from statements by officials and orders by those in authority and that is this: despite innumerable remarks that disease has been brought about or will result from the refuse, no scholar of the original records refers to any mention of rats. One can scarcely imagine that people liked having them around for they would foul food, eat it and cause indoor disturbance in the structure of dwellings and would be regarded as vermin. If they were present they would undoubtedly have fed upon the offal and scraps and one complaint about refuse must surely have been that it sustained rats in some numbers. Yet there is no mention of these rodents in this connection. It is not proof of their absence and it may be argued that rats were so much a part of everyday life as to be taken for granted. Yet I find this difficult to believe for two reasons. Firstly, things were commented upon with some precision and when there were murrains even the deaths of sparrows were noted. Secondly, if rats were present, when bubonic plague arrived in 1348 there would have been heavy rat mortality, a fact well known and commented upon by people in endemic plague areas, and as this would have been the first occurrence of rat plague experienced by the English then that fact alone would have been an important feature of the times. So far as I can find there was no occasion when this was recorded in the British Isles in 1348–50, a point made by Henschen (1966) who also drew attention to the fact that there was no mention of mass deaths among rats during the Justinian plague or in the great Moscow epidemic of 1770.

There is evidence from India that plague-infected rats wander in the open in a moribund condition although this spectacle was not observed in the Colombo epidemic of 1914 (Philip and Hirst, 1917). These authors found few dead rats in the open and no conspicuous evidence of an epizootic despite the high proportion of plague-infected rats. They believed that the carcasses were easily hidden because of the structure of the roofs of native dwellings. As we have seen in Egypt (p. 107) dead rats were found within the fabric of a building but they were also picked up from the floors of most rooms.

Taking the evidence reviewed in this and the preceding chapter, one must conclude that the environment was unlikely to have been adequate for the widespread build-up of large populations of a warmth-loving species so dependent upon buildings. In large urban and trading centres, especially ports, more permanent populations might be envisaged, topped up, as in modern times, by rats coming ashore from ships and being transported inland in merchandise.

CHAPTER SEVEN

Fleas and plague

All cases of bubonic and septicaemic plague in man are begun by the bite of an infected flea which has recently left the body of a dead rodent host. The majority of pneumonic plague cases probably arise secondarily from primary bubonic plague although man to man droplet transmission may occur directly. Primary pneumonic plague from rodent to man without flea contact is rare. Thus the biology of the flea vector is of great importance in plague outbreaks and was extensively studied by the Plague Research Commission. Their findings provide us with a guideline of the physical factors necessary for flea breeding and plague transmission and the basic biology recorded by the Commission stands little altered today. By extrapolation from the past we may be able to judge whether alleged epidemics of plague could have taken place on the likelihood of fleas being able or unable to operate in certain climatic conditions.

Fleas live on birds and mammals and show modifications to an ectoparasitic way of life similar to lice. The body of the flea is flattened laterally; this enables it to move through fur with greater ease and to leap to a new host, the back legs which provide the force in the jump being enabled to operate in the vertical plane. The eggs of fleas, unlike those of lice, are laid loosely on the body of the host and they drop off and hatch on the floor of the burrow or in the nest of the host rodent. The larvae which hatch out have stout body hairs and biting mouthparts and feed on organic detritus. They usually pass through two larval moults, by which time they are fully grown and ready to attach themselves to a suitable host.

Adult fleas take blood from their host with their piercing and sucking mouthparts and this is their only food. Most fleas can survive on blood from several species but some are more restricted. The rabbit flea, for example, *Spilopsyllus cuniculi* cannot breed until the flea feeds on a pregnant rabbit or its newborn young (Mead-Briggs and Rudge, 1960); certain substances in the rabbits' blood during the last part of pregnancy stimulate maturation of the flea (Rothschild and Ford, 1966). The rat flea, *Xenopsylla cheopis*, however, does not appear to need the hormones of the host. Flea larvae eat a variety of organic materials provided they are dry and finely divided. For most flea larvae the blood of the host is an important food item and they obtain it by eating the faeces of the adult fleas. Because the latter feed to excess, almost totally undigested blood passes out of the anus.

Climate is very important for fleas and, unlike lice, which are little affected by climate, they often undergo seasonal cycles. This is because part of the flea life cycle is passed away from the host and they are therefore less protected from fluctuations in the climate. In temperate latitudes adult fleas are most abundant in the warm parts of the year, both larvae and eggs developing only within fairly narrow ranges of temperature and humidity. As an example, the eggs of three common fleas have the following tolerance ranges:

Xenopsylla cheopis (rat flea):	13°C to 34+°C
Pulex irritans (human flea):	8°C to 34°C
Nosopsyllus fasciatus:	5°C to 29°C

The larvae of these three species show similar but narrower ranges of tolerance. Under *optimal* conditions the life cycle of a flea may be completed within three weeks. However, if the climate is unfavourable or starvation occurs, the various stages of development may be prolonged (Bacot, 1914).

Because climate, particularly temperature and humidity, is so important in the maintenance of flea populations on mammals and within their burrows, it is therefore a major factor in the epidemiology of plague. Even before the Plague Research Commission began work it was known that epidemics only occurred at certain times of the year in certain parts of India, there being a periodicity in the number of cases at any particular place. With this in mind the optimum conditions for fleas were examined and found to be as follows:

1. a relative humidity of .70 and over and a temperature of between 18.3°C and 29.4°C were the most favourable conditions for the hatching of flea larvae;
2. on the other hand, very high temperatures, i.e. over 29.4°C and dry air would reduce the period of infectivity, the length of the fleas' life and also the larval production of the flea.

These points were borne out by the seasonal prevalence of plague in India at that time. The number of plague cases was reduced when the temperature rose to a daily average of 28°C and the relative humidity fell. In Bombay the most severe epidemic was in the early part of the year, whereas in May to July, when the daily average temperature was 35°C, cases were few and sporadic. In Poona, 80 miles away but at an altitude of 2000 feet, epidemics occurred in the last part of the year, the dry weather of March to May producing few or no cases.

Other basic flea research was conducted by Bacot (1914) working in England on the influence of temperature and humidity using artificially regulated atmospheres and also by the Department of Public Health in Egypt (Petrie and Todd, 1923). The latter, for various reasons, converted humidity data into the equivalent vapour pressure deficiencies (V.P.D., in millibars). This, they claimed, had the advantage over the relative humidity figure of giving a more exact measurement of the drying capacity of the air. The Egyptian workers concluded that:

1. for *Xenopsylla cheopis*, temperatures from 20°C to 25°C and V.P.D.s from one to ten millibars were most suitable for its development at all stages;
2. the higher the temperature and the V.P.D. (a high deficiency indicating excessive dryness of the air) the shorter the period of survival of adult fleas when kept unfed.

When the Egyptian workers tested these conclusions against epidemiological information relating to the seasonal prevalence of plague in six Indian cities – Bombay, Poona, Belgaum, Lahore, Nagpur and Rawalpindi – tabulating deaths, temperature and V.P.D. grouped in fortnightly periods, the results did not agree well with their findings, the discrepancies being most noticeable in the data for the up-country stations. However, the agreement improved when the plague incidence for any fortnightly period in the epidemic season was compared, not with the corresponding temperature and V.P.D. figures, but with those of successive preceding fortnightly periods up to a limit of four to six weeks. The general conclusion arising from this modification was that the extent of the disease at any moment in the epidemic period was dependent upon atmospheric factors in operation some six weeks before, and not upon the strictly contemporaneous weather conditions. They then pointed out that even in places with diverse climates, the mean temperatures and V.P.D.s that prevailed six weeks before the peak of the epidemic fell within a range that varied from 20°C to 25°C and from one to ten millibars. There was, then, an optimum mean temperature and V.P.D. within these limits for the spread of the disease, the lag between optimal conditions and epidemic peak being due to the time taken for the complete development of *X. cheopis*. Since the Indian epidemic curves were of plague *deaths*, the lag period would include an interval of about 12 days that elapsed between the time of infection by the flea and the human death.

Analysis of some Indian data showed that for places where there were wide diurnal temperature variations, e.g. Lahore, the correlation was less good than for places such as Bombay where the range of variation was smaller. Thus, hourly temperature variations during the day should perhaps be considered because they would exert a changing influence which would either stimulate or curb flea development (Petrie and Todd, 1923). A comparison of the number of favourable hours could then be compared with human plague data. The Egyptian team made an approximate analysis for Lahore in the light of these ideas and found that the results confirmed their hypothesis.

At the beginning of this century some tropical cities had few plague cases whilst others had severe outbreaks. Colombo, for example, despite the opportunities of all tropical ports at that time for importing plague, was never badly infected. Two, possibly three, factors contributed to this state of affairs: the mean monthly temperatures varied from 26.1°C to 28.7°C and the flea average was low. It was also thought that the high incidence of *Xenopsylla astia* instead of *X. cheopis* explained the relative immunity of Colombo (Hirst, 1927–8). It was thought in India that the prevalence of *X. astia* was associated with a low incidence of plague. On Java, the port of Surabaya (mean temperatures 26.0°C to 28.1°C and with a low flea average), was immune compared with Malang in the hills at 400 metres above sea level where plague was prevalent.

In Egypt, plague was seen to diffuse from the south to the north of the country across the four divisions, these being, from south to north, Southern Upper Egypt, Northern Upper Egypt, the Delta and the northern ports. The normal temperatures and V.P.D.s for the month preceding that of maximum plague prevalence in these same four divisions respectively were: 14.9°C, 20.5°C, 22.1°C and 23.8°C and 7.9, 11.7, 9.8 and 7.9 millibars.

The Plague Research Commission (1908) charted human plague deaths, temperature and relative humidity for each available year from 1897 to 1906. They concluded:

> 1. that the rise of the epizootic and consequently of the epidemic depended upon a suitable mean temperature somewhat below 29.4°C and over 10°C (plus sufficient susceptible rats and a sufficient number of rat fleas);
> 2. that the fall of the epizootic and epidemic was determined by a high mean temperature: 29.4°C and above (plus a diminution in the total number of susceptible rats and an increase in the proportion of immune to susceptible animals together with a diminution in the number of rat fleas).

They noted that in Poona the epidemic decreased despite the temperature being suitable and speculated that some other factor must operate to bring about this decline. Further investigations by the Commission in Poona (Plague Research Commission, 1910), Belgaum (Plague Research Commission, 1910a), the Punjab (Plague Research Commission, 1911) and the United Provinces (Gloster and White, 1917) led them to the belief that the hygrometric state of the atmosphere had an important bearing on the diffusion of the disease. The charts which they constructed in the Poona and Belgaum enquiry showed a strong correlation between flea prevalence and relative humidity. They inferred that when the mean daily temperature fell within the limits 16°C to 27°C the flea prevalence varied directly with atmospheric humidity. In the Madras Presidency plague diffused feebly, the Commission considering that the unfavourable conditions of heat and drought acted as a barrier to the transportation of infected rat fleas. They had already shown that the effects of drought and a high temperature were lethal to rat fleas separated from their host.

Brooks (1917) concluded that there was a critical saturation deficiency for each range of temperature. At 26.7°C the critical saturation deficiency was around 0.30 inch. The important point in relation to outbreaks was that at lower temperatures epidemics would be suppressed by a higher degree of deficiency and at higher temperatures a lower deficiency was sufficient.

An examination of the epidemic curves throughout the year in those places where plague was seasonal shows that there were two types of epidemic curve for human plague. The data for Bombay, Calcutta and Hong Kong give symmetrical curves; in Bombay not only the epidemic curve was symmetrical but also that of the epizootic (for 1906) and of the flea variations (for 1907). The investigators explained the portions of the curves representing the epizootic and epidemic periods by the rat flea variations, which were mainly a function of temperature, as the V.P.D. was rarely unsuitable. The non-epizootic and non-epidemic seasons were accounted for by the high temperatures which reduced the numbers of fleas by being detrimental to the developmental stages and shortening the life of infected fleas whose valve of the proventriculus was inoperative.

Where the fall is more rapid than the rise, as in Lahore, Nagpur, Cawnpore and Lucknow, the curves were asymmetrical. No epizootic curves were available for comparison. In this class of curve the flea variations were again the principal factor but in addition there was a further modifying feature which the Egyptian workers suggested resided in the wide range of diurnal temperature variations typical of those localities. They suggested that during some part of the day the temperature rose so far above the optimum as to exert a retarding influence upon the transference of the infection to rats and people by shortening the life of infected fleas.

The essential difference in the two types of curve results from the effect of high temperature on the course of the epidemic, the point in time when such temperatures operate determining the two patterns. In the symmetrical curve, e.g. Bombay, the amplitude of the diurnal temperature wave is smaller than in the up-country cities and, whilst excessive temperatures are also lethal to infected fleas, the effect is seen towards the end of the epidemic period. In an asymmetrical curve, e.g. Lahore, the effect appears at the time of maximum plague prevalence. Whether the factor was temperature alone or V.P.D. or some combination of the two, it produced its effect within a short period, acting directly on the flea vector of the disease.

Returning to the European situation, Shrewsbury (1971) points out that in addition to great heat and drought, which shorten the life of blocked fleas, frosty weather in temperate latitudes causes *X. cheopis* to hibernate. According to the work of Bacot (1914) temperatures below 7.2°c were fatal to all stages, save the adult, of *X. cheopis*. Shrewsbury goes on to say that modern knowledge of the bionomics of this flea explains why in medieval England epidemics of bubonic plague usually erupted towards the end of spring, rose rapidly to a peak of intensity in late summer or early autumn, collapsed or declined sharply with the arrival of autumn frosts, and were extinguished in or remained dormant throughout the winter months. As the epidemic disease of 1348–9 was active in all seasons it would imply that either it was not plague or, as is usually assumed, bubonic changed to pneumonic plague when cold weather occurred.

Shrewsbury says that seasonal periodicity was a notable feature of medieval plague epidemics in Europe, being brought about by the effect of the climatic conditions upon the rat flea population, the fleas flourishing in a temperature range of 20°C to 25°C together with some dryness of the atmosphere. He points out that a period of good breeding weather for fleas will produce an increase in population of *X. cheopis* in one month (three weeks according to Pollitzer, 1954) and this will lead to a human outbreak if the disease is already epizootic amongst the rats. There is, then, a lag between the onset of the most favourable flea-breeding conditions and the first human cases, a feature commented upon at length by the Egyptian and Indian research workers. This lag period does not appear to have been evident in Europe when the epidemic arrived in 1347 and onwards.

The climate of the British Isles and Europe must be taken into account in this analysis of factors capable of sustaining plague or of being detrimental to its progress by way of the flea vector. From 6000 B.C. to 3000 B.C. occurred the warmest climatic period since the Ice Age. Warmth-loving trees grew and, from botanical evidence, the prevailing summer temperatures in Britain were estimated to be 2 to 3°C above present normal values. Following this, the climate deteriorated generally, although there were some better periods in between, with increased storminess and finally the rapid advance of glaciers in the Alps and the re-birth of many of them. After 900 B.C. there was the development of the cool, moist 'sub-Atlantic' climatic period, a time when the former ways across the Somerset levels and other English lowlands became flooded and water transport was used. The size of Alpine glaciers in western Austria had increased by 500 B.C. from a small fraction of their area around 1000 B.C. to more like their maximum size attained around A.D. 1650.

In Roman times the climate was probably not very different from what it is today. Some recovery followed and there was a warm epoch which culminated between A.D. 1000 and 1300. The climatic deterioration of the late Middle Ages was evidenced by great storms which occurred in the period 1250–1570 and by sea-floods which occurred in 1170–8, 1240–53, 1267–92, 1374–7, 1393–1404 and 1421. A cold epoch which was the coldest since the Ice Age and often known as the Little Ice Age began about 1300 and culminated between about 1550 and 1700–1850 (Lamb, 1966). In Norway this climatic deterioration is said to have so reinforced the effects of the Black Death that many of the farms in the exposed uplands, in coastal districts and in the north lay waste and remained so for 200 years. However, if the climate was so poor, with lowered temperatures, it is difficult to see how the Black Death could have been able to operate bearing in mind the needs of *Rattus rattus* and fleas. There was some slight amelioration in these harsh years around 1500 and a tendency to go back to the plough around 1530, a reversal of the process of conversion from open-field agriculture to sheep that had been going on for a long time.

TABLE 5

Calculated winter and summer temperatures from A.D. 1100– A.D. 1850

Period	Average temperature, °c, for winter months of December, January and February.	Average temperature, °c, for high summer months of July and August.
1100–1150	3.5	16.5
1150–1200	4.2	16.7
1200–1250	4.1	16.7
1250–1300	4.2	16.7
1300–1350	3.8	16.2
1350–1400	3.8	15.9
1400–1450	3.4	15.8
1450–1500	3.5	15.6
1500–1550	3.8	15.9
1550–1600	3.2	15.3
1600–1650	3.2	15.4
1650–1700	3.1	15.3
1700–1750	3.7	15.9
1750–1800	3.4	15.9
1800–1850	3.5	15.6

Data from Lamb (1977)

This cold era was followed by warmer temperatures in the twentieth century. Utterström (1955) supports Lamb's account, saying that in the 70 or 80 years before the Black Death the climate began to change. It was reported that the cold increased and that both Alpine and polar glaciers advanced. There was heavy rainfall and the level of the Caspian Sea rose. The cultivation of cereals in Iceland and the vine in England almost finished and in the uplands of Provence and in Denmark the growth of wheat was reduced. In Table 5 is shown the calculated average temperatures for the winter months of December, January and February and for the high summer months of July and August for 50 year periods from 1100 to 1850 (Lamb, 1977). This clearly shows a fall in the winter and summer averages from 1300 onwards and from what has been said earlier about the optimum conditions for flea hatching it can be seen that at no time between 1300 and 1850 was the average July–August temperature suitable for this purpose. Despite the higher summer averages for the earlier part of the period (1100–1300), not even then did the

TABLE 6

Mean temperatures (°C) for the years 1931–60

City	Jan.	Feb.	Mar.	Apr.	May	June	July	Aug.	Sept.	Oct.	Nov.	Dec.	Year
Aberdeen	2.4	2.8	4.5	6.6	9.0	12.0	14.0	13.6	11.7	8.8	5.6	3.7	7.9
Manchester	3.3	3.4	5.9	8.2	11.7	14.2	15.8	15.6	13.6	10.3	6.8	5.1	9.5
London	4.2	4.4	6.6	9.3	12.4	15.8	17.6	17.2	14.8	10.8	7.2	5.2	10.5
Plymouth	6.2	5.8	7.3	9.2	11.7	14.5	15.9	16.2	14.7	11.9	8.9	7.2	10.8

Mean temperature (°C) of inland England for the years 1931–60

Jan.	Feb.	Mar	Apr.	May	June	July	Aug.	Sept.	Oct.	Nov.	Dec.	Year
3.4	3.9	5.9	8.4	11.4	14.6	16.2	16.0	13.7	10.1	6.7	4.7	9.6

Data from Manley (1970)

temperature become generally high enough, being only 17.4°C. Clearly, calculations of this stated precision for times so long past will be criticised, no matter how carefully they have been calculated, yet there is considerable agreement amongst climatologists and biologists about the detail. Perhaps it is prudent to also examine the climatic data for recent times when, after the mid-nineteenth century, the temperatures began to improve. Manley (1970) reviewed the English climate and Table 6, from data in Manley, gives the mean temperatures for the years 1931–60 for Aberdeen, Manchester, London and Plymouth as well as the mean temperature of inland England during the same period. It is seen that in no month does the mean temperature reach 18.5°C, the lowest point in the optimum hatching range of temperatures. Mean temperatures hide maxima but this is not a serious objection to their use. If they occur only occasionally and for short periods they will have little effect on the mean: if they occur for longer periods of time then the higher mean will show this.

Taking the four cities in Table 6 the climate data in Manley for the same period show that in no month did the maximum reach 18.5°C, July being the highest with 17.9°C and August second highest with 17.5°C. Average daily minima for the same months were 10.1°C and 9.6°C. This illustrates what is typical of temperature in Britain, namely that whilst it may reach flea-hatching temperature on occasions within a month it will also during that same month fall to low levels as well. Isolated hot days are of little importance in producing a constant high level of flea breeding.

If we turn to examine summer maxima and minima for the other cities we see that for Manchester the maxima of 18.5°C and above occur in June (18.7°C), July (19.9°C) and August (19.7°C) but the corresponding minima are 9.7°C, 11.7°C and 11.5°C. In London the equivalent temperatures, with minima in brackets, are: June 20.3°C (11.4°C), July 21.8°C (13.4°C), August 21.4°C (13.1°C) and September 18.5°C (11.0°C). In Plymouth the two months in which average daily maxima reached or exceeded 18.5°C were July, 19.0°C (minimum 13.0°C) and August, 19.3°C (minimum 13.0°C).

Relative humidity in Britain is never likely to be a factor limiting flea breeding. Table 7 gives the relative humidity per cent averaged through the 24 hours for the four cities whose temperatures we have considered. Only in London during the summer months does the relative humidity fall to a level around or only slightly above the threshold of 70 per cent relative humidity. This is the time and place showing the highest temperatures although the mean for the months is still not high enough to promote hatching.

Figure 8 (after Arléry, 1970) shows the mean temperature (°C) in July over western Europe for the period 1931–60. The whole of Britain, northern France, the Low Countries, north Germany and Denmark, in addition to an area in southern France, lie below 18.0°C.

Shipley (1911), discussing the prevalence of rat fleas, pointed out that whilst *Xenopsylla cheopis* was apparently cosmopolitan it did not flourish in

TABLE 7

Relative humidity (%) averaged through 24 hours for the period 1931–60

City	Jan.	Feb.	Mar.	Apr.	May	June	July	Aug.	Sept.	Oct.	Nov.	Dec.	Year
Aberdeen	88	84	84	81	82	81	83	84	84	86	88	89	87
Manchester	89	89	82	78	74	77	79	81	82	84	86	86	85
London	88	84	79	73	72	70	72	75	80	85	88	89	81
Plymouth	89	87	85	81	81	82	85	85	85	86	87	89	87

Data from Manley (1970)

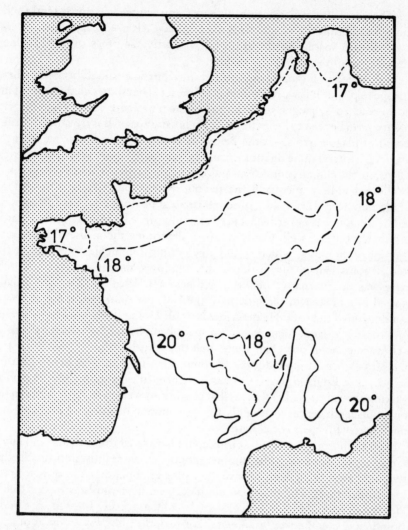

Fig. 8 Mean temperature (°C) in July over western Europe, 1931–60 (after Arléry, 1970)

temperate and cold climates but was the commonest of the rat fleas of warmer countries. This point is worth bearing in mind and may be of importance when considering the reasons for the failure of the Suffolk plague outbreak of 1910–12 to extend further (Chapter 9).

From a climatic point of view, therefore, the British Isles and some of northern Europe does not appear to provide adequate conditions for most of the time to sustain regular seasonal outbreaks of flea-borne bubonic plague even in summer, let alone the winter months. Shrewsbury says that north of the Thames valley it is doubtful whether any winter was consistently mild enough to permit the plague fleas to continue their predatory activities. Yet some disease spread northwards and was active at times other than high summer, as for example in Yorkshire.

As an added point in the question of the climatic unsuitability of northern Europe to plague it is worth looking at Figure 3. That shows all the parts of the world reached by plague since the end of the nineteenth century and the vast majority can be seen to be in the warmer climatic zones. It is true that there is a record of plague arrivals in the British Isles this century but as we shall see later in Chapter 9 these did not expand far compared with, say, South Africa.

Despite the climate, conditions indoors could have been made favourable if dwellings had been adequately heated but there is some evidence that on the whole they were very cold. Although fire had obvious qualities for cooking and heating, it was nevertheless used carefully since buildings made of wattle and thatch burned well. Coulton (1949) describing the medieval scene says that one of the things which would pinch us most immediately would be the cold. Rooms had ill-fitting doors and windows, mostly unglazed, so that there was no alternative between darkness and open air. The fire usually burned in a brazier in the middle of the hall, the smoke escaping as best it could through the roof. He describes how, in Montaigne's *Voyages*, when he goes to Switzerland, he notes with a special emphasis how the rooms are so well warmed with porcelain stoves that one actually takes off one's hat and one's furs when sitting indoors and comments that in mid-sixteenth-century France, as in England, warm clothes were needed even more indoors than in walking abroad. It is likely, then, that conditions were even more bleak in the mid-fourteenth century, certainly for the common people, and probably not much better for their social betters.

Even supposing that *Rattus rattus* could have lived in the thatch and fabric of peasant houses during the summer months, it seems most improbable that it would have been able to survive the winters in buildings so exposed to the low temperatures. The thatch would have been the best place for rats to live but even that would have been extremely cold, especially since the fire in the room below could never be too large for fear of setting fire to the roof.

Such few studies as have been made show that the flea numbers on rats in the British Isles are low compared with those in tropical plague areas. Shrewsbury says that a rat can harbour 17 flea species (he presumably means that 17 species of flea have been recorded from rats the world over) and the flea population of a rat may total several score, although he gives no reference to support this figure. The average number of fleas per rat in the Suffolk outbreak was one (range 0.1–3.3 per rat), a figure which compares unfavourably with the data from Kôm Ombo, Egypt, in 1911 (Table 8). It was said that one of the chief features of the severe epidemic of 1911 was the high degree of infestation of houses with *Xenopsylla cheopis*.

Pointing out that only two of the rats' species of flea, the Asiatic rat flea,

TABLE 8

Flea infestations on the three rodent species at Kôm Ombo, Egypt, during the plague epidemic of 1911

Habitat	Average number of fleas per rat		
	Arvicanthis niloticus	Rattus norvegicus	Rattus rattus
Houses only	22.1	32.6	–
	6.0	14.5	–
Fields	11.2	22.0	–
Feluccas	–	29.4	14.0

Xenopsylla cheopis, and *Nosopsyllus (Ceratophyllus) fasciatus* are constantly capable of acting as vectors of plague, Shrewsbury says that the former was the more dangerous vector and was *almost certainly exclusively responsible* for the great medieval epidemic of bubonic plague in Europe. This is pure supposition although it is true that where *known* epidemics of bubonic plague have occurred originating from an epizootic amongst rats, then *X. cheopis* has been mainly involved.

Hirst (1927–8), Roubaud (1928) and Girard (1946) have all claimed that *X. cheopis* was common in past centuries in Europe and was therefore able to play the main role in the frequent epidemics of plague. The fact that *X. cheopis* subsequently disappeared from Europe was attributable to the replacement of *Rattus rattus* by *Rattus norvegicus*, a rat which is supposed to be a less suitable host for this flea. As Pollitzer (1954) says, this is a fascinating hypothesis but one that is difficult to accept. *Xenopsylla cheopis* in fact has no specific predilection for *R. rattus* and is abundant in Manchuria where *R. norvegicus* is the predominant rat species.

If *X. cheopis* can then establish itself in the cold of Manchuria it might be argued that it could have done so in Europe where the winters are much less severe. But the *X. cheopis* colonies which have been found in modern Europe have almost without exception been sited in the basements of steam-heated buildings where even in winter the temperature was high enough to enable this flea to develop and survive. *X. cheopis* prefers a warm climate and because of this it must be considered doubtful whether the temperatures of the houses of medieval Europe were suitable even in summer, let alone winter. In Manchuria the species survives because of the heating methods which are commonly found in houses. These have wide, elevated platforms made of brick and because they are used for sleeping as well as for living purposes, are kept warm day and night with the aid of flues. *X. cheopis* is also frequent in Korea where identical living conditions probably account for its frequency.

Because it is so widely distributed the origins of *X. cheopis* are in doubt but

Jordan and Rothschild (1908) considered that its true home was the Nile Valley and pointed out that it occurred in all warm climates whilst Jordan (1938–9) believed that it originated in Iran, Iraq and their adjacent countries.

The fleas of commensal rodents which are present in any given locality are often unevenly distributed, showing preferences for what Toumanoff and Herivaux (1948) called 'micro-sites' which are favoured by particular fleas although the suitability of these sites will be largely governed by the suitability of the microclimate prevailing in them.

X. cheopis is mainly found infesting commensal rodents living in buildings, unlike such species as the palaeoarctic *N. fasciatus* and also *X. vexabilis hawaiiensis*. In a favourable climate such as India, Uganda and the southern U.S.A., *X. cheopis* is found more in the commercial than the residential quarters, particularly in premises where foodstuffs, especially cereals, are stored and handled and also in cotton mills and warehouses (Hirst, 1933–5; King and Pandit, 1931). Cotton is most suitable for harbouring *X. cheopis* and in the Cumbum Valley rat nests containing cotton had a higher incidence of this flea than did ordinary nests.

Macarthur (1926) suggested that the feeding habits of flea larvae may modify the behaviour of adult fleas. The larvae of *Ceratophyllus fasciatus* and others require blood for their development which they obtain from the faeces of the parent. Thus, the necessity of providing the larvae with food confines the adults to the nest. But fleas like *X. cheopis* have larvae which do not need blood and therefore the adult has no reason to desert the host. Such a flea is therefore more dangerous from the point of plague transmission because the adult fleas would be, for example, on a rat feeding in a grain store. These fleas carried by the rats might lay large numbers of eggs and the larvae would feed on the grain and other debris and mature, thus producing a dense flea population. As a corollary to this he points out that a flea census on rats infested with *X. cheopis* and *C. fasciatus* would give misleading figures regarding respective numbers on rats because a large proportion of *cheopis* would be found on trapped rats whereas most of the *fasciatus* would have remained in the nest. The dry conditions found in granaries and warehouses where cereals are handled favour *X. cheopis* because such places are prone to rat infestations and the cereal debris forms a suitable nourishment for the larvae.

Even in tropical climates such as Ceylon and southern India the indigenous *X. astia* has showed a more widespread distribution than *X. cheopis* although even that flea was sometimes restricted to residential quarters. It was occasionally predominant in places where rice was stored or handled. It is said that *X. cheopis* was more prevalent in underground burrows than in nests found in ceilings or roofs although in the Cumbum Valley this flea did not exhibit a preference for any particular level. Most, but not all, evidence indicates that *X. cheopis* has an affinity for rats living underground rather than for those sheltering on the higher levels of houses. The same seems to be true of *N. fasciatus*.

Although we speak of 'infected' fleas these ectoparasites[11] are not actually infected with plague in the true sense of the word. They harbour the plague bacilli in the gastro-intestinal tract where multiplication occurs in the stomach or proventriculus. One of the factors which makes *X. cheopis* an efficient vector is the high infection rate. This can be studied under laboratory conditions by allowing fleas to feed on experimental rodents in which bacteraemia has reached a high degree. Eskey and Haas (1940) showed that even under optimal conditions only about one third of the fleas became infected (Table 9). There are marked differences between the different flea species in the infection rate. In fleas examined by Eskey (1938a) the infection in *X. cheopis* was 66 per cent compared with about 25 per cent in the case of *N. fasciatus* and some others and ten per cent in *L. segnis*. Eskey (1938b) held the view that the different infection rates in the various flea species might depend on differences in their feeding habits. If a flea species fed at long intervals it would be less likely to obtain a meal during the time its host had many bacilli in the blood. *Xenopsylla cheopis* is a voracious feeder, a fact which might explain the high incidence of infection in the species.

TABLE 9

Relationship of host septicaemia to percentage of fleas becoming infected after feeding

Degree of septicaemia in hosts (guinea-pigs)	Number of fleas fed	Percentage of fleas plague-infected
10 or more organisms/field in smear*	439	32
2–10 organisms/field in smear	457	29
1 or less organisms/field in smear	546	25
Smear negative, cultures strongly positive	469	17
Smear negative, cultures slowly positive	344	10

*This would represent a high degree of septicaemia

Clearly, the number of bacteria taken in per meal is important. The average volume of a flea's stomach was long ago calculated to be 0.5 mm^3, therefore a flea taking in rat blood containing 10,000 or more plague bacilli per millilitre would take into its stomach at least 5000 bacilli. However, Douglas and Wheeler (1943) estimated the volume of *Xenopsylla cheopis* stomachs and showed that the capacity was much smaller than the estimations of the Plague Research Commission. In no case did a flea, even in a small, half-filled stomach, ingest as much blood as had been claimed and the earlier average of 0.5 mm^3 was 16 times larger than the more modern estimate. It was estimated that 66 per cent of plague rats in Bombay had more than 10,000 bacilli per millilitre of blood either before or immediately after their death and that approximately 50 per cent of the fleas collected from these rat bodies harboured *Y. pestis*.

Further, the retention of plague bacilli by the fleas is a factor making some species more effective vectors. Phagocytosis[12] was known to be increased by a rise of temperature up to 40°C (Plague Research Commission, 1908a) and under experimental conditions a rise in temperature of about 8°C between the limits of 24°C and 32°C doubled the rate at which bacilli disappeared from the flea gut. Work by Ledingham (1908) showed that phagocytosis of some bacteria at 18°C was only about one-fourth to one-fifth of that at 37°C. In this respect *X. cheopis* comes out well again because it retains the bacilli. Douglas and Wheeler (1943) showed that approximately 60 per cent of infected *Diamanus montanus* and two per cent of *X. cheopis* were able to free their alimentary canals of *Yersinia pestis* after a single infectious blood meal. In *D. montanus* this process took 24 hours but in *X. cheopis* it required more than 48 hours.

Before the bites of plague-infected fleas are infectious, the infection has to undergo a period of incubation in the flea. In experiments carried out by Eskey and Haas (1940) this period varied from five to 130 days, differing in length in fleas of the same species and among different species. The time which is needed for the incubation is important in determining the efficiency with which different species of fleas transmit plague: the shorter the incubation, the more rapidly will the disease be transmitted. Of all the species they tested, *X. cheopis* was found to transmit plague in the shortest time after becoming infected.

This, then, covers the main points of the relationship of fleas to climate and to the bacilli of *Y. pestis*. One further thing to consider is the question of the part played by fleas when they are transported to other areas. This transport may be by their host in the case of shipborne rats, in merchandise such as bales of cotton or sacks of rice, by humans either on their persons or in their baggage or on a transport vehicle. The movements of fleas by their own efforts are quite considerable: for example when starved they can make vertical leaps of c. 10cm (4 inches) and when gorged with blood can leap c. 7.5 cm (3 inches). They can jump horizontally just under 15 cm (6 inches) and can walk up a vertical sheet of glass for c. 20 cm (8 inches). *Pulex irritans*, an almost cosmopolitan flea, misnamed the 'human flea', can leap vertically 19.5 cm (7¾ inches) and horizontally 33 cm (13 inches).

From their experiments the Plague Research Commission concluded that the spread of infection at a distance was effected by infected fleas carried either on a person or in the bedding of travellers who had either lived in plague houses or had visited them. It was the opinion of the Commission that such fleas were not directly responsible for causing human plague (even travellers carrying flea-infested baggage were able to escape infection) but produced rat plague in the places to which they were transported. The vital information in this sequence is how long an interval elapses between the release of a few fleas into the local rat population and the epizootic which in turn leads to the first human cases.

In Egypt, Petrie and Todd (1923) came to the same conclusions as the Plague Research Commission although in Java the importance of the transportation of plague-infected fleas by travellers was doubted, only two *X. cheopis* and one *Stivalius cognatus* being found among the ectoparasites collected from the clothing or baggage of 56,790 travellers who had left the partly plague-affected province of Malang. Even the clothes of a group of 1829 persons, among whom there were 393 plague patients, yielded only seven *X. cheopis*. In the opinion of workers in Java the transport of fleas by travellers was a minor factor in the spread of plague in that country and Pollitzer (1954) says that one ought to agree with the opinion of Hirst that, in general, a spread of flea-borne plague through travellers is of comparatively limited importance.

The transport of infected fleas in goods, especially in raw cotton, gunny bags, rags and hides is generally agreed to be of great importance in the spread of plague. There has, however, been plenty of debate on just how far the infection can be carried by such fleas. Hirst (1931) said that the available evidence pointed to the fact that when an overseas source of infection was only a few days away, an infected flea might be readily transferred directly in grain from the port of origin to the port of entry but otherwise it would be inferred that a plague epizootic had occurred among the rats aboard ship. The link between the ship epizootic and the shore rats or the rats of the lighters into which cargo was loaded or unloaded could be a plague-infected rat but was much more likely to be a plague flea. Citing the case of plague passage from Rangoon to Colombo, 1234 miles (1985 km) distant, Hirst said that the transference of infected fleas all the way from Rangoon to Colombo without their feeding on ship rats *en route* was theoretically possible but the sea voyage was about two days too long to favour this mode of spread. This, bear in mind, was with steamship travel so it is worth thinking back to the original route by which plague is supposed to have travelled from the Crimea to Europe. In Chapter 3 I calculated that the distance from Caffa to Messina was about 1600 miles and to Genoa 2200 miles.

After examining various evidence of plague transport, Pollitzer (1954) concluded that it was unlikely that long-distance transportation of infected fleas played a generally important role in plague dissemination. If this were the case, then instances of ship-borne transference of the disease would have remained frequent in spite of the measures now widely adopted to eradicate rats on ocean vessels. He pointed out that, in fact, instances of long-distance spread of plague through the maritime traffic had almost ceased and concluded that there was little doubt that *infected rats, rather than infected fleas, carried in consignments of goods* (my italics) were responsible for this dissemination of plague.

As I have mentioned in earlier chapters, various flea species as well as *X. cheopis* can transmit plague and a few notes are appropriate here on some others:

Nosopsyllus fasciatus: this species is of European origin and according to Jordan (1948) it had become almost cosmopolitan but was still not present in some countries. Outside its normal range it is usually found in ports and adjacent districts. It was, according to Jordan, rare in India.

Leptopsylla segnis: also called *L. musculi*, this flea, like *N. fasciatus*, is another palaeoarctic species which has become almost cosmopolitan.

Pulex irritans: this flea is known as the human flea but it has a wide range of hosts including pigs, goats, foxes, badgers (Jordan, 1948), and is said to occur on commensal rats, dogs, cats, hares, many rodents, wild cats and rabbits. It originated in the Old World and is now almost cosmopolitan.

Ctenocephalides felis & *Ct. canis*: also of palaeoarctic origin but now almost cosmopolitan. These two species occur on cat and dog respectively, their specific hosts, and also on commensal rats and other rodents. Both will attack man and may become serious pests in houses (Pollitzer, 1954).

Other arthropods may be involved in plague transmission although in a minor way. Human lice, *Pediculus humanus capitis*, can transmit plague to guinea-pigs and positive cultures have been obtained from plague-infected bed bugs, *Cimex lectularius*, for up to 35 days. The bugs also infected laboratory animals with plague by biting them. The lice of plague rats can harbour *Y. pestis*. The lice of ground squirrels can also harbour plague and these could transfer plague to experimental animals. A mite, *Laelaps echidninus*, on *Rattus norvegicus*, has conveyed plague from rat to rat and, finally, it is known that ticks can harbour *Y. pestis* but there is no further information on that point.

CHAPTER EIGHT

The rate of spread in modern epidemics of plague

It is my principal aim in this chapter to examine the spread of plague amongst the human population of rural and urban areas in those modern epidemics where we can be sure that plague was present and to compare our findings with those outbreaks of the disease in the Middle Ages which are thought to be bubonic plague. In a consideration of spread on land crucial factors are the speed of spread of the rat epizootic and localised human movements. Transoceanic passage of plague must also be taken into account because it enables us to pinpoint the source of an infection and its time of arrival in a country and may also show how long the organism can survive in a ship-board rat population.

When the plague bacillus in the blood becomes active, producing a fatal septicaemia in a rodent, the blocked fleas transfer the disease to other rodents of the population and the epizootic is under way. The speed with which it spreads throughout the rodent population will depend upon the chances the fleas have of contacting other rodents. It is probably more than a chance happening that bubonic plague is so closely associated with rodents because they frequently exist at high densities, a factor which enables the transfer of fleas and bacillus to be facilitated. Such a method of transfer would be inappropriate for solitary living species. Although seriously affected by plague man is of little importance in the maintenance of the disease whose continuance depends upon sufficient numbers of resistant rats in a population or, in the case of sylvatic plague, of resistant species within a geographical area.

It is of vital importance to know how fast an epizootic in a rat population will spread across that population from a pre-existent focus. A distinction has to be made between such a continuous expansion of infection, called 'intramural' spread by Gill (1928) where, for example, plague spreads from one section of a city to another, and spread at a distance, which has been called 'metastatic' spread by observers in Java. Intramural spread from rat to rat may be an extremely slow process. The Plague Research Commission (1907) gave

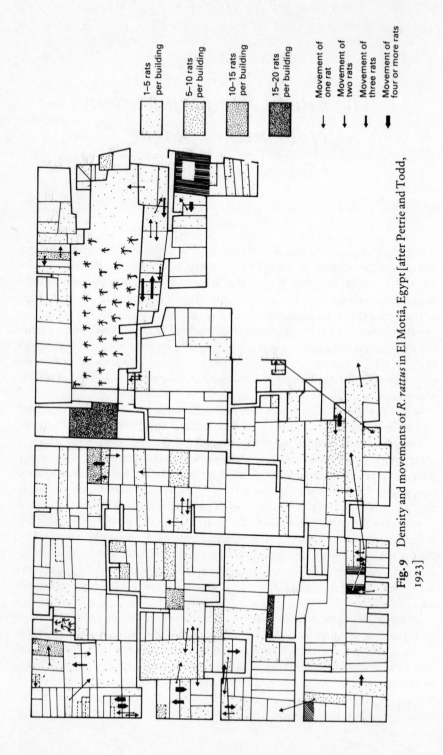

Fig. 9 Density and movements of *R. rattus* in El Motiâ, Egypt [after Petrie and Todd, 1923]

1–5 rats per building

5–10 rats per building

10–15 rats per building

15–20 rats per building

Movement of one rat

Movement of two rats

Movement of three rats

Movement of four or more rats

an instance where a rat epizootic took six weeks to travel 300 feet. The spread of the epidemic was not centrifugal but irregular, although when the investigators put guinea-pigs into the houses they said that the result led to the conclusion that the infection spread peripherally from the focus in Soliwada section of Sion village in India.

The extent to which individual rats move about depends on the species of rat and the habitat in which it lives. As *Rattus rattus* is the only species under consideration as a plague carrier in the Black Death then all modern comparisons will be with the same species. Generally, the extent of rat movements is exaggerated and in practice it is seen that under the normal daily routine rats move quite small distances.

In a plague epidemic in El Motiâ, Egypt, in 1912 some of the earliest attempts at discovering rat movements were made (Petrie and Todd, 1923). The town had 1291 occupied houses, 279 of them in one experimental square. From the viewpoint of rat movements these dwellings were interesting because they were in groups of contiguous houses with few alleyways and only one block of houses was totally separated from the rest by an alley. A total of 341 *R. rattus* was individually marked. The investigators concluded from the recaptures that the movements of the rats were limited, most of them being oscillations between contiguous houses (Fig. 9) and representing sorties for food from nests and burrows situated in the foundations of walls common to adjoining houses. Only one *Rattus rattus* reached an adjoining square; this rat covered in all 250 metres, but in several stages, so far as one can make out from the account taking 15 days in the process. Thus, an epizootic commencing in the interior of a square in El Motiâ would receive a check when it reached the boundary.

This was an important study because, so far as I can discover, it was the first time that rats had been individually marked, systematically re-trapped and their movements recorded. The finding that the broader streets acted as barriers to rat movements is of great practical importance in rodent control and the epidemiology of plague. El Motiâ is warm at all times of the year (the coldest month, January, being 11.1°C and the hottest, July, 28.0°C so that, presumably, factors other than temperature prevented the rats moving far. In the cold, wet British climate movements beyond the house in which they might have lived would be expected to be even rarer.

Even the Brown rat moves surprisingly small distances. In Baltimore it was found that in urban areas 71 per cent of adult males and 77 per cent of adult females were recaptured within 40 feet of the point of original capture. On a farm the movements were similarly limited (Davis, Emlen and Stokes, 1948; Davis, 1953). In Cyprus, Watson (1951) found that 67 per cent of male and 77 per cent of female Black rats moved less than 50 yards; rarely did animals move more than 100 yards.

In Hawaii, Tomich (1970) studied the movement patterns of *Rattus rattus* in coastal fields of sugar cane and in adjacent uncultivated land where the climate was weakly tropical (average annual temperature 22.2°C with a mean range of approximately 4°C) and food supplies continuous throughout the year. The average distance between captures for rats repeating capture in less than a month was 90 feet for male *Rattus rattus* and 73 feet for females. In this same study of *Rattus rattus* living under what would appear to be optimal conditions the density was surprisingly low and was higher in uncultivated land, with a maximum of ten and a minimum of one per acre, than in a cane field where comparable figures were three and none. Due to reaping and general disturbance the latter was an unstable habitat.

Finally, writing in 1899 on rats and plague, Aitken had this to say, 'The Indian house rat is not fond of crossing open country, where it would be at the mercy of any owl, cat or mongoose that saw it. It trusts for safety to concealment and to its agility in climbing. In the Deccan it seems very unlikely that infection could ever be carried from village to village by rats unless the interval were very short.' Unless there are exceptional circumstances, such as the total destruction of the habitat, rats move little and thus, as already mentioned, the spread of an epizootic can be a slow business.

Objective figures of rat populations in towns have not borne out the widely held impression of high rat density. For example, in El Motiâ the 279 houses of the experimental square had an average of 1.2 rats per house and roughly the same number of *Acomys* per dwelling although, as we have seen from India (Chapter 6), houses in Belgaum had higher rat populations. Shrewsbury (1971) maintains that the distribution and density of the rat population governs the distribution and intensity of human plague. He says that the rodent density is decisive because no serious outbreak of bubonic plague can take place in a locality supporting only a small or widely dispersed rat population. He further argues that as *Rattus rattus* is dependent upon man, because of food and cover, then the rat density must have been related to human density. Furthermore, the human disease must have been proportionate in extent to the density of the human population and since that was uneven so was the incidence of bubonic plague uneven. Shrewsbury is insistent that the density of *Rattus rattus* is of great importance in engendering an epidemic of bubonic plague. For this to happen the rodents must be present in such numbers that the density of the rat population is high enough to enable *Y. pestis* to be distributed rapidly over the area of the epidemic by haphazard rat-contacts. The mere presence of the rat, he avers, is not enough to do this.

All this is probably true although no one has ever been able to quantify the necessary density. Because the effects of plague in the nineteenth and twentieth centuries have been perhaps greatest in parts of India where human overcrowding and a high rat population go together, this may be the area where the necessary optimum conditions outlined by Shrewsbury are found. As I have said earlier, there are no grounds to support the belief that *Rattus rattus* was widespread in the British Isles, although it was perhaps present in a few urban centres. This at once demolishes the idea of a well-distributed rat population away from dwellings and without that rat population bubonic plague during the Black Death would have needed some other agency to spread it across the extensive rural human population.

Accounts of the medieval pandemic have all emphasised the speed with which the disease proceeded and in Chapter 4 I have given some estimates of its speed of passage in western Europe. Simpson (1905) pointed out that the Black Death was distinguished by its rapid spread and destructiveness and said that never before had plague shown such diffusive qualities. In marked contrast to this the progress of the disease in India had been slow; in fact during the first three years, as pointed out by the Indian Plague Commission, the disease was not able to extend and take a hold of the country in such a way as seriously to affect the ordinary death rate. He points out that this slow diffusion is one of the most constant characteristics of plague, as evidenced by the fact that the Great Plague of London took six months to travel from St Giles' to Stepney.

In Asia, especially China and perhaps some parts of India, plague was already present from the past in sylvatic form. This needed activating and the spread could therefore be quite different from that in a region where plague had never been before and to which it came in rats for the first time. It is to such areas that I next turn because they represent a direct parallel with plague in western Europe in 1348–50.

South Africa makes the ideal starting point because there is no record of plague in the country before the early part of 1899 and the documentary account of its spread is accurate. Most of the following is from the historical summary of plague in South Africa by Mitchell (1927).

In the latter part of 1898 an epidemic of plague occurred in Tamatave, Madagascar, and a vessel, the *Gironde*, from that port which was reported to have plague cases on board was refused entry by the Portugese on arrival at Lourenço Marques and returned to Madagascar. In late November 1898, mortality of rats in a certain quarter of Lourenço Marques occurred but it was never known whether they had died of plague.

In mid-January 1899, four cases of bubonic plague in male Indians from the same house occurred in Lourenço Marques. A fifth case was found at Middelburg in the Transvaal on 6 February, about 200 miles inland from Lourenço Marques, in an Indian who had come to Delagoa Bay on a ship from Bombay on 5 January. Although there were no plague cases on board, the vessel was put in quarantine for 21 days and the 127 Asiatics, including the one who subsequently developed plague, were eventually allowed to land on 26 January. The man stayed in Lourenço Marques until 31 January when he left for Heidelberg, Transvaal. He became ill at Komatipoort and was taken off the train at Middelburg. A sixth case was found in a man at Lourenço Marques on 7 February. All six cases were bubonic and three of them died.

In early 1900 a family from Mauritius arrived at Durban. Two or three weeks later one of the sons became ill with high fever and a groin bubo. Plague was diagnosed and the case was fatal. Three or four days before becoming ill the son had opened the last of their trunks which they had brought from Mauritius. It was thought that an infected flea had travelled with clothing as plague then existed at Mauritius. In October 1900 plague occurred at Izeli, a native area, with 13 cases of which four died. There were no domestic rodents and few veld rodents in the area and none of the latter showed sickness or mortality. It was believed that the infection was brought by infected rats or fleas in forage from the Cape Town docks where an epizootic was causing rat deaths at the time.

The most serious epidemic in South Africa took place in Cape Town and its neighbourhood in 1901. On 1 February 1901, an unusual mortality of rats in part of the docks was seen and was found to result from plague. This section of the docks had been in the hands of the military from the beginning of the Anglo-Boer War in September 1899 and contained large stores of grain and forage which had been imported from several South American ports, notably Rosario, Buenos Aires and Rio de Janeiro where plague was present. Enquiries revealed that the rat mortality had been present for six months since August 1900 and during the week before plague was diagnosed two suspicious deaths had occurred. Investigation revealed that the rat population throughout the dock area and that part of the town adjoining it was widely infected with plague. According to Mitchell, soon after this an exodus of rats from the dock area occurred and carried the infection practically throughout the town and suburbs. There is no more information on the actual details of this unusual occurrence. If it took place it probably resulted from a massive cleaning-up operation in the dockyard food stores, which was a likely event once plague had been discovered in the rats.

A severe epizootic and human epidemic followed and lasted through 1901 with 766 cases being known, of which 371 died. Eighty per cent of the cases were bubonic and in most of them plague-infected rats were present in the dwelling or where the patient worked. It was seen that pneumonic cases usually originated from a bubonic case with lung complications and that such infection diffused rapidly: if the case was not promptly discovered and isolated then the infection soon spread to the immediate contacts.

In Port Elizabeth in April 1901, plague-infected rat bodies were found in the harbour area and despite attempts to localise the outbreak by erecting rat-proof fencing, the epizootic spread and was followed by human cases. This outbreak was different from that in Cape Town where both epizootic and epidemic were of the explosive type. In Port Elizabeth, both in rats and man the disease was of the slow-spreading, smouldering type and later in its course there were considerable intervals between successive cases; for example, in late 1902, as many as 82 days elapsed between successive human cases.

Mitchell gives some interesting and important observations about the nature of the epizootic: 'Rats in one block of stores would die in small numbers over a period of several weeks, whilst rodents in adjoining blocks remained healthy; on the latter at last becoming infected, the same process of slow diffusion would go on. In the great majority of cases in man infection was traceable to rodents.'

It is worth bearing in mind at this point that at the end of 1901 it was three years since the first cases of plague had been identified at Lourenço Marques. In this period there had been 786 cases of human plague and 377 deaths, the majority occurring in the Cape Town epidemic. During the same period of time the Black Death in Europe had proceeded from its first arrival on the toe of Italy in December 1347 to the north of Norway by December 1350 (Langer, 1964) and had reduced the population of Europe by about 24 *million*, from 84 million to around 60 million, the greater part of the mortality occurring in the initial impact. In South Africa, however, the disease after three years and, in all probability, multiple introductions from steamships coming from the plague-infected ports of the Orient, India and South America, was still only present in a few ports.

Between 1901 and 1905 rat epizootics and human epidemics occurred in several places. At Knysna, on the coast in Cape Province midway between Cape Town and Port Elizabeth, the town was badly rat-infested and a severe epizootic ensued but only one human case resulted. Here the plague epizootic extended to veld rodents (striped mice, *Rhabdomys pumilio*) in the dense woods around the town and there was heavy mortality among them with infected carcases at places 12 and 18 miles from the town.

During this period plague-infected rodents, without human cases, were found at many places. There was some evidence to indicate that railways acted to spread infection in forage or crated goods and on one occasion an apparently sick rat was caught leaving a goods truck at a town over 100 miles from Port Elizabeth from which port the train had arrived. The rat was plague-infected.

Up to 1912 there was, either prior to or concurrent with human epidemics, an infection of the rats. These had introduced plague at the ports and spread the disease to other centres, the great majority of human cases being traceable to murine infection. Beginning in 1914 it was suspected that plague had moved into the sylvatic phase because a series of outbreaks occurred on farms in remote rural areas, notably in the Cape Midlands in 1914–15, and although there was reason to believe that these had their origin in veld rodents it was not until 1921 that it was proved (Mitchell, 1921). From then onwards the history of plague in southern Africa is the expansion of sylvatic plague over great areas inhabited by gerbils who form the chief sylvatic focus.

Two important facts emerge from the first 14 years of plague experience in South Africa. The first is that, despite heavy rat infestations, plague did not sweep through even the coastal cities in the way that reports tell of it doing in fourteenth-century Europe. By the end of 1912 the total number of cases was 1750 with 986 deaths. Between then and 30 June 1926, many if not most of the cases recorded had their origins in veld rodents and by June 1926 the number of cases recorded since the first in 1899 was 2568, 1505 of whom died. The proportion of cases dying, 58.6 per cent, was high but by no means unusual in the days before antibiotics. It is important to distinguish between plague case mortality and the mortality due to plague in the population as a whole. Because of the high case mortality in the pre-antibiotic era there is a tendency for this figure, e.g. 60 or 70 per cent, to be accepted as the proportion of people in the total population dying of plague and hence it is often assumed that if plague was present then, automatically, 60 or 70 per cent of the population could be expected to die of the disease. At no time since the current pandemic began has this been true anywhere in the world.

The second point of note is that, despite the occurrence of pneumonic plague in South Africa on several occasions, there was never a countrywide epidemic resulting from these foci. There has been a general acceptance by many writers on the Black Death that winter cases were pneumonic and that the speed of spread of that pandemic could only be explained on the assumption that the pneumonic form predominated or even excluded bubonic. Even when, following the deaths of ten or 12 native farmworkers from pneumonic plague on a farm about 100 miles inland from East London, the rest of the natives on the farm stampeded and carried the infection to neighbouring farms and surrounding districts, there was no rampant outbreak, only a few further cases. The most serious phase in this focus occurred early in the epidemic. The first 26 cases were all in immediate contacts, all were pneumonic and only one survived.

The rate of spread of plague, both in the murine and the sylvatic phases, is

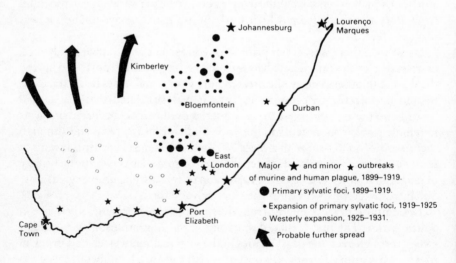

Fig. 10   The spread of plague in southern Africa (after Davis, 1948)

well documented in South Africa and Figure 10 shows the progression of the disease in that country. Table 10 presents comparisons of rate of spread in epidemics in this pandemic and during the fourteenth century.

TABLE 10

Rate of spread during the Great Pestilence of 1347–50 and the plague pandemic of the late nineteenth and early twentieth centuries.

Country	Rate of spread	
France 1347–8		
Marseilles to Carcassone	5 miles per day	
Carcassone to Bordeaux	1½ or 3 miles per day	
Marseilles to Avignon	1½ miles per day	
Avignon to Lyon	2 miles per day	
Marseilles to Paris	2½ miles per day	
England 1348–9		
Melcombe to Bristol	1½ or 4 miles per day	
Bristol to London	2 miles per day	
	Murine	*Sylvatic*
South Africa *1899–1925*	8–12 miles per year (perhaps aided by trains)	c. 20 miles per year
India	?	?
North America 1901–40	?	8 miles per year
England Suffolk 1906–10	4 miles per year	—

The importance of the concurrence in time and place of the epizootic and the epidemic was shown in Egypt in 1912 in Abnûb Town (Petrie and Todd, 1923). The town had 16,000 persons yet despite a considerable rat infestation (413 *R. rattus* in one infected square, averaging, for 355 rats, 11.5 fleas per rat) there were only 48 cases, all either bubonic or septicaemic. The epidemic lasted from 1 January to 9 April and spread through the squares of the town lying parallel to the Nile bank. The spread of the infection did not suggest that the disease invariably progressed by contiguity from house to house because it was interrupted in places.

During the same period Qûs Town, with 15,000 persons had 82 cases of which 51 were bubonic, 16 had no obvious buboes and 15 (18.3 per cent) were pneumonic. There were 61 deaths (74.4 per cent of cases). This epidemic was slow to start, unlike medieval epidemics: the first case was noticed near the east side of the town on 14 January 1912 and several dead rats and two plague-infected rats were picked up or caught in a grainstore in the house of the patient. It was 43 days before the second case occurred, at the north-west corner of town, and five members of the patient's family also contracted bubonic plague. The source of infection could not be traced to the first focus. From 26 February to 9 March, ten cases were reported from the West side but there were no more cases there until the middle of April. On 28 February, a death occurred in a house in the first infected square. Most of the cases were subsequently from the east quarter of the town but the distribution of the bubonic cases was so irregular as to suggest the presence of at least four isolated epizootic areas. The research workers were of the opinion that the creation of apparently independent foci of rat and human plague in a town like Qûs was attributable to the transportation of infective rat-fleas by persons who either inhabited or visited infected areas of the town although these persons may or may not suffer from plague in consequence. Nevertheless, as in South Africa, in both Abnûb and Qûs the disease did not reach the alleged proportions of medieval plague nor spread beyond the confines of the town. These Egyptian towns were discrete, fairly large units and in size corresponded closely to fourteenth-century Bristol.

A situation more akin to that of rural medieval England existed on the Kôm Ombo estate on the Nile bank, 520 miles south of Cairo. Of recent origin, it consisted of 25,000 acres scattered over which were 29 hamlets with a total population in 1912 of 12,831 and an average of 250 people per hamlet. There was, then, a population density of 0.5 people per acre. Plague began in January 1911 and according to the official account was severe (Petrie and Todd, 1923). They said that the outbreak which followed had no parallel in Egypt in modern times. Many of the hamlets became infected, and the spread of the disease was so rapid that hundreds of people fled in panic to their native districts leaving some of the villages almost deserted. Some of these persons were suffering from plague and were traced to towns and villages farther north. 357 plague cases with 237 deaths (66.4 per cent) were recorded from January to the end of April but these figures were considered an underestimate. Although the report has a section on the sequence of infection in the hamlets it disappointingly provides information from only two of these. In one, with 920 people, there were eight bubonic and septicaemic cases in a month and in another, with 364 persons, 20 unspecified cases. Severe as this epidemic undoubtedly was, it still represents a plague mortality of only 1.85 per cent of the total population of Kôm Ombo.

The 1907 census of Egypt gave a total population of the cultivated areas, excluding nomads, of about 11.2 million. The population density was 939 persons per square mile (362 per square kilometre) with Aswân district having the highest density of 640 per square kilometre. There were 3,581 villages, most of them with less than 10,000 inhabitants, but the criterion of a village was clearly quite different from that used in medieval Europe. In the 20 years from 1899 to 1919, 14,783 *cases* of plague were notifed: that is, 739 per annum on average (approximately 0.007 per cent of the population) or 65.9 *cases* per 100,000 people per annum. As Petrie and Todd pointed out, the numbers are small when compared with India where the *deaths alone* in each of the first ten epidemics in Bombay ranged from 10,000 to 20,000 in a population of nearly one million. Furthermore, despite the panic and movement of people in Egypt to escape plague, some escapees taking plague with them and dying elsewhere, there was, taking the country as a whole, no widespread outbreak.

In Hawaii it was clearly demonstrated that plague was slow to spread to places even with direct railroad connections, in contrast to its rapid spread by sea. Plague first appeared in the Chinese section of Honolulu on 12 December 1899 from Hong Kong or Japan (Eskey, 1934). Honolulu operated as a feeder port to other island ports and from there plague spread quickly to the islands. The pattern of cases in Honolulu was as follows: after the first case there was a gap of 12 days and then 17 cases occurred in the last week of December 1899. In January 1900, there were 35 cases, in February, ten and in March, nine, making a total of 71 in three and a half months, a mild introduction and similar to the pattern in South Africa.

Although plague has become endemic in Hawaii there has never been any severe outbreak but, as Gross and Bonnet (1951) pointed out, with periodic recrudescence of human plague and the continued presence of plague in both rodents and rodent fleas, constant vigilance was necessary. The region is favourable to rats of various species, the yearly mean temperature at sea level is between 22°C and 24°C, varying seasonally by only one or two degrees, with plenty of food and cover for rats and it is curious that despite such conditions plague has never been severe in the islands.

Plague entered North America for the first time during this pandemic and some human cases occurred. In March 1900 the first case of human plague in the United States was recorded in San Francisco. Between 1900 and 1904 there were 121 cases with 113 deaths (93.4 per cent case mortality) at San Francisco and during a second outbreak in 1907–8 there were 160 cases with 78 deaths. Twelve cases were also reported in Oakland, across the bay from San Francisco (Eskey and Haas, 1940). It was generally accepted that the rats of San Francisco were infected through the medium of oriental shipping some time before the discovery of human cases, although rat infection was not demonstrated until 1902. Many plague-infected rats were found in Seattle at irregular intervals from 1907 to 1917. Unlike South Africa, the spread from domestic rats to local rodents, in this case ground squirrels, was rapid and the latter were reported as having died in great numbers in the vicinity of San Francisco Bay in 1903. Five years later plague infection of ground squirrels (*Citellus beecheyi*) of this region was proved bacteriologically and investigations during 1909–10 showed that plague was established among ground squirrels of nine counties to the south of San Francisco Bay. The spread of plague to many species of endemic rodents has been well documented by

Eskey and Haas (1940) and has little part in the present discussion, except to show how permanent is the sylvatic focus. When they wrote in 1940, plague had persisted in some of the coast counties from the time of its introduction until then, being continuously present in the two San Francisco Bay counties of Alameda and Contra Costa until 1928 in spite of active campaigns to eradicate it. Other counties had remained plague-infected for nearly 30 years, the region constituting this original and persistent enzootic focus being practically the entire Coast Range Mountains from San Francisco south to Los Angeles County.

After the initial outbreaks there were two subsequent epidemics in seaports. In 1919 a pneumonic epidemic of 14 cases with 13 deaths occurred in Oakland, California, the initial case being a man who became ill a few days after shooting and dressing ground squirrels for food. The last outbreak (prior to 1940) in a Pacific coast port appeared at Los Angeles in 1924. During this epidemic, which was secondary to an epizootic among rats, there were 32 pneumonic cases with 30 deaths and seven bubonic cases with four deaths. Except during the early years an important aspect of plague in the western States was the comparative absence of domestic rat infection. This was due to the scarcity and uneven distribution of rats in the West and their almost total absence from vast areas of the intermountain region. This absence of rat plague was an important factor in the comparative infrequency of human infection. Nevertheless, spread of human plague was slight even when there were pneumonic cases.

The evidence from India, where the most severe effects from plague have been seen suggests, despite the high mortality, that with all the crowding, high rat and flea numbers, plague did not run riot in the way it is said to have done in the fourteenth century. The work of the Plague Research Commission presents adequate information on the course of the disease in small to medium sized communities of the size predominant in medieval England. Some, called villages in India, would have greatly exceeded most medieval settlements outside the large towns.

In a village of 950 people it was seen (Plague Research Commission, 1907) that the duration of the epizootic amongst the rats was two months and, as mentioned earlier (p. 133), diffusion amongst the rat population was slow. Within a house the infection lasted ten days in rats from the first plague rat to the last, that is providing there was no re-infection from outside.

The villages in this study (Plague Research Commission, 1907) had suffered annually from plague for many years so that although it was not a new situation the course of each epidemic could be charted. One or two interesting ideas about diffusion were introduced when a study of one village revealed that, during an epidemic, 61 per cent of the cases acquired their infection outside the village. They commented: 'There is no evidence to show that the disease spread from man to man when infection was imported into the village by sick persons. Persons living in the same room as the sick did not contract the disease.' In bubonic plague this is true and as we have seen from South Africa, North America and Egypt, even though pneumonic plague may diffuse rapidly to immediate contacts, no widespread epidemic followed. The exception to this is the Manchurian epidemics which will be outlined and discussed in Chapter 9.

Another aspect of diffusion is the role of the so-called human flea, *Pulex irritans*. Ell (1979) considered that the evidence from medieval texts pointed to transmission by the human flea as the mode of plague infection during the European epidemics of the fourteenth and fifteenth centuries. He could find no satisfactory evidence to support a spread involving *Rattus rattus* and *Xenopsylla cheopis* nor any support for the minority opinion that pneumonic plague operated. His evidence in favour of human flea transmission is not very convincing and the very point that plague was regarded as being infectious by interpersonal contact might suggest evidence of some other diseases. Another point to consider is that if plague was transmitted by human fleas without a rat reservoir, it is difficult to explain recrudescence of plague in the same human population after a period of quiescence. Ell makes one significant point from his reading of the many texts and that is that 'animal mortality during epidemics of plague was noted, but the rat never mentioned'. He quotes from documents which state that the plague struck dogs, cats, chickens, cattle, asses and sheep and points out that the mortality of animals from plague was noted, but that the rat mortality necessary to postulate rat-borne plague was not described.

He observes that interhuman transmission via the human flea is the predominant mode of spread in North Africa and the Middle East. The position there may not be so clear cut, however, and it is worth examining the conclusions of the authors quoted by Ell on a study of plague in Iran. Baltazard *et al.* (1960) adduced evidence showing that epidemics of bubonic plague in Kurdistan, where there were no domestic rodents or 'liaison' rodents, were due to interhuman transmission by the human flea, beginning with rare cases of plague contracted in the fields. They pointed out that such interhuman plague, originating in villages, tended to die out rapidly because of the scanty population of villages, the long distances between them and the paucity and poverty of the means of communication. Such might have been the fate of fourteenth-century plague in human fleas and there was almost certainly no sylvatic reservoir then. The Iranian workers then go on to point out that when imported into an urban area with a dense human population, 'plague immediately becomes the terrifying disease it was during the Middle Ages'.

Baltazard (1960) elaborates further on this theme, stating that plague can become epidemic only when there is interhuman transmission by human ectoparasites 'as is shown by the existence in the Middle East of plague epidemics in the absence of rats' (in the previous paper he made the point that such plague died out rapidly) 'and the non-epidemic nature of the disease in

India, despite the presence of rats and of *Xenopsylla cheopis* in numbers never reached in any country or at any time' (we have no basis for such a statement, especially regarding time). He goes on, 'The great slaughter caused by plague in olden days was all due to transmission by human ectoparasites', (this is pure supposition) 'but the duration of the epidemics must have been dependent on the existence of a large murine background. Indeed, if any proof of the presence of *R. rattus* in the ancient world is required, it is supplied by the very existence of plague'. If, as I believe the evidence shows, there was little or no murine component, this method of transmission could not exist. Furthermore, if, as Baltazard suggests, a large population of *R. rattus* was necessary it might be equally well argued that it and its own flea was perfectly capable of initiating and sustaining a plague epidemic.

Wu, Lien-Teh *et al.* (1936) were of the opinion that human parasites, whether fleas, bed-bugs or lice, were only of practical importance in the spread of human plague under peculiar circumstances and, unlike the rat fleas, were unable to lead to widespread and persistent epidemics of bubonic plague.

The Indian workers experimented with *Pulex irritans* and obtained three successful transmissions out of 38 experiments, the fleas having previously been fed on septicaemic rats. They concluded from this that transmission of infection from man to man by means of the human flea was probably a very infrequent occurrence. From what is known of the multiplication of plague bacilli in the flea it seems clear that spread by the human flea would have to depend on the septicaemic phase being prevalent and this is infrequent in epidemics. As most cases are bubonic with low bacilli numbers in the blood – numbers inadequate to make fleas biting them infective – it thus seems very unlikely that extensive man to man transmission by the human flea would take place. I have earlier (Chapter 7) said that *Pulex irritans* has a wide range of hosts, including rats, and the remains of a fifteenth-century rat from the Baynard's Castle site in London have been recovered with this species of flea on its fur. The commentary on this find (*New Scientist*, 1982) suggests that the presence of the human flea is the reason why plague spread so quickly and was so severe and that this flea was at least partly responsible for the spread of the fourteenth-century epidemic in London. The author suggests that *P. irritans* flitted fairly freely between rats and people. It may have done but from what I have just said about its capacity as a plague transmitter it may not have been as capable a vector as is suggested.

Martin (1911) suggested that if the plague bacillus developed greater infectivity, with perhaps diminished toxicity leading to a higher degree of septicaemia in man, this would permit of direct transmission by human fleas. Bubonic plague could then be independent of the rat and spread directly from man to man. He produced no evidence to support this idea. It would be a pronounced shift in the biology of the disease (one for which there is no evidence) and, to take but one objection, the speed of the medieval epidemic could not be explained by flea transfer in a sparse human population.

Burnet (1962) says that as the Black Death developed its activity, it is almost certain that transmission by flea from rat to man was very largely displaced by man to man transmission, either by fleas, or directly when the disease took on the pneumonic form. He claims that there is distinct evidence that in the winter of 1347–8 the pneumonic form was dominant, while in the following summer nearly all victims contracted the bubonic form. Even assuming that rats were present there is little evidence, either from contemporary writing in England or the information from modern epidemiology, that this shift in spreading mechanism took place and to say that it is almost certain can only be guesswork. Further, Burnet says that there is a tendency for plague contracted from burrowing wild rodents to take the pneumonic form, while the disease derived from rats is almost always bubonic and he quotes as evidence the fact that in modern times the only great epidemics of pneumonic plague have been in Mongolia and Manchuria, where the tarbagan is the important reservoir. This certainly seems to be the case but whatever doubts we may entertain about medieval plague in Europe we can be fairly certain that there was no sylvatic reservoir which, according to Burnet, would be necessary to provide the amount of pneumonic plague that he suggests was present. It is true that non-murine rodents may produce human pneumonic plague but we must not forget that this form may, as in South Africa and Egypt, arise also from murine infection.

The role of human movements must be taken into account as a factor aiding spread and this has already been referred to on various occasions. The Egyptian research team assessed this and pointed out that if it were possible to ensure that the human agent remained wholly passive the infection would proceed in a regular manner outwards from a centre, the first focus. The Plague Research Commission (1907) replaced the evacuated human population in an infected village with guinea-pigs and showed a uniform progression amongst the experimental animals. In Egypt the movements of people spread infection, such movements being greatly assisted by the railway which in 1912 had 1,481 miles of track and carried 28 million passengers. There were several cases of sick people being taken off trains: they had plague and were fleeing from infected villages. Other features assisting plague spread in Egypt were the *mulids* (fairs of a semi-religious character) and markets, there being 180 of the former per annum which lasted altogether for 1,300 days and attracted 750,000 visitors. The Egyptian work pattern caused regular temporary migration resulting from the lack of cultivation in the southern provinces of Upper Egypt in the summer months.

It is apparent from these certain examples of plague that the spread of the disease, even when pneumonic, is less rapid than is supposed and that on no known occasion has it acted at anything approaching the speed of the great disease of the fourteenth century. Nor has it produced, even in India, a similarly high mortality. The examples I have given from the current pandemic have all possessed one salient feature in common: the presence of a well-established rat population in which an epizootic has been responsible for the subsequent human epidemic. This fact is fundamental to extensive plague epidemics and, I believe, goes some way to explaining the slower speed of spread in modern outbreaks. As Shrewsbury has said, 'In every instance of an epidemic of bubonic plague in history, an epizootic of the disease in a domiciliary rat population must have preceded and progressed concurrently with the human disease.' Coupled with the rapidity of passage and the high mortality of the Black Death, my doubts about the existence of extensive medieval rat populations add strength to the argument that some disease other than bubonic plague must be sought as the agent of the fourteenth-century epidemic in Europe.

CHAPTER NINE

Twentieth-century plague in Britain and a general consideration of pneumonic plague

It may surprise many to learn that plague has been present in the British Isles in the twentieth century, yet when we consider the maritime traffic between Britain and those countries in whose ports plague was already established, it would perhaps have been more remarkable if it had not reached these islands. The interesting feature is that despite multiple introductions, with the disease in one rural area becoming extensive, and with several cases in various ports, plague did not become established as it has done in many parts of the world. Neither, interestingly enough, did it establish itself in the rest of northern Europe.

Ships represent the greatest danger of introducing plague, mainly by means of rats and fleas in the cargo, and in the years 1896 to 1901 plague was diagnosed in several crew members of ships from the East, especially India, and there were some deaths. In all, there were 82 known cases on 54 ships coming to England, five of them on a ship which had turned round in Hull and was returning to South America, and of the 82 17 were fatal. The peak years were 1899 to 1901, with 74 of the cases in that period (Low, 1902).

It is clear from the events at two ports that plague came ashore. In Cardiff in January 1901 a man died of plague. He worked at a flour mill at Cardiff docks and two weeks before his illness began it was noted that rats had been dying in some numbers in the mill and the deceased man had handled some when taking them to be destroyed in the mill's boiler furnace. There was a similar case in the following month when, at another flour mill, a man who had conveyed dead rats to the furnace became ill. Plague was not found in this case but the fact that rats had died in the mill gave grounds for suspicion that the disease had been introduced. Plague bacilli were obtained from a dead cat at one of the mills.

In the autumn of 1900 in Glasgow there were 36 plague cases with 16 deaths in the few houses to which the infection was confined but no plague was found in a few hundred rats examined. In 1901, five cases occurred in a rag store nearby. Rat plague was found and later five human cases were confirmed in a hotel. Plague-infected rats existed in the basement and there was an extensive epizootic in the neighbourhood. In August 1907, two plague cases occurred in a rag store and although there was no plague in rats nearby a single infected animal was found beneath a police station a mile away. It seemed likely, therefore, that rat plague had probably been going on for at least seven years, with little effect on human health (Hirst, 1953).

Plague outbreaks also occurred at Liverpool, Hull, Bristol and London but they were small, sporadic, and limited to a small area. At Liverpool in 1901, eight of 11 cases died and there was a suspicion of interhuman transmission.

All these foci were in ports, the traditional route of entry in most plague-infected countries and in no case was there evidence of extensive spread. However, in rural Suffolk a little later (H.M.S.O., 1911) there was evidence of plague being much more widespread as the following account shows. I have dealt with the events in some detail because they represent the only occasion there has ever been to study plague in a rural situation in the British Isles and because a clear appreciation of them is important in assessing past epidemics believed to have been plague.

The area of the outbreak

On 2 October 1910, the medical officer of health of Samford rural district, Suffolk, notified to the Local Government Board on Public Health and Medical Subjects four cases of what was described as 'pneumonic plague' from Freston. This hamlet was situated four miles south-south-east of Ipswich in an area of farmland bounded on two sides by the Rivers Stour and Orwell to the south and north respectively (Fig. 11).

The houses in which the cases occurred (A) were about one mile from the River Orwell and almost three miles from a point on the river called Butterman's Bay (I). It is possible that this latter locality may be of importance in the occurrence of plague in the area. At the time of the outbreak Ipswich was an important port receiving grain-laden vessels from various parts of the world. Because boats of deep draught were unable to proceed direct to Ipswich Docks they stopped at Butterman's Bay to be lightened, some of the grain going to Ipswich and elsewhere by other craft. The Samford area was thinly populated, almost everyone working in agriculture.

History of the illness

Three of the sick people came from one cottage, the middle one of three, and were the father, mother and a nine year old girl, one of four children of the family. The girl was taken ill on 12 September 1910 and died on 16 September, the mother and father being taken ill on 21 and 26 September respectively and dying on 23 and 29 September. A fourth patient, a 43-year-old woman who lived a quarter of a mile to the north (B) was taken ill on 26 September and died

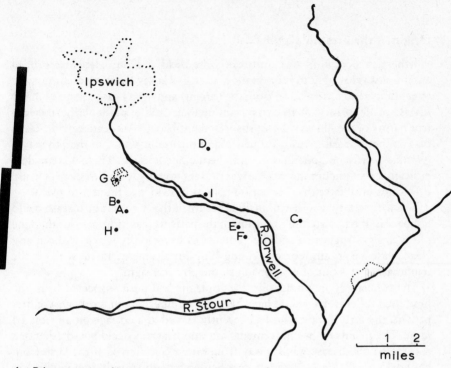

A – Primary cases of human illness at Freston
B – Secondary cases of human illness at Freston
C – Primary cases of human illness at Trimley
D – Secondary cases of human illness at Nacton
E – Primary cases of human illness at Shotley
F – Secondary cases of human illness at Shotley
G – Wood at Freston in which the first rat dead of plague was found
H – Wood at Holbrook in which the first hare dead of plague was found
I – Buttermans Bay

Fig. 11 Localities in Suffolk in which outbreaks of human illness occurred and positions in which certain plague-infected rodents were discovered

on 29 September. She had nursed the mother of the first household on the night she died, 23 September. The child aged nine, who was the first person to be taken ill, had returned some eight days previously from the cottage of some relatives approximately three miles to the east.

The illness was short and there was probably lobular pneumonia, a characteristic feature of pneumonic plague, in two if not three of the four cases, in addition to diarrhoea and vomiting in three of the patients. Subsequent bacteriological examination of cultures from the lungs of some of the patients left the bacteriologists and doctors in little doubt that the organisms were those of plague, a point of view that was later to be reinforced by the finding of undoubted rodent plague in the vicinity. The evidence was therefore very strong that the four people died of pneumonic plague.

Origin of the Freston plague outbreak

All the sick people in this outbreak were dead and buried before official attention was brought to bear on the matter. Because of this it was impossible to get first-hand information from the patients and in any case the speed of the disease made it difficult to cross-examine them in life, particularly since the true nature of the illness was not suspected until later. The death certificates in two of the four cases read 'Influenza and pneumonia' and in the other two 'Gastric catarrh and pneumonia' and 'Septic pneumonia'. There was no clear indication that pneumonic plague was present nor any reason to suspect it and it was not until later that the various pieces of evidence fitted into place.

The first oddity was the anomalous nature of the attacks. The disease could not be classified. Also, the condition of the patients was more serious than the physical signs suggested and the patients became rapidly worse without any clear evidence of any corresponding lung involvement. In most cases the temperature was out of proportion to the physical signs.

The official report points out that if plague had been suspected from the first, then fuller notes would have been made, especially in regard to the first patient, the girl of nine who had recently stayed at a cottage on an isolated farm. The details of her movements are important in deciding whether she contracted the disease whilst away from home. She arrived at the farm from her home on 28 August and left on 4 September, apparently in good health. Whilst there she played in the harvest fields but the fact that there were no cases from this area would indicate that the origin of her infection was not from her holiday site and subsequent enquiries revealed no illness in the cottage where she stayed nor in other cottages on the farm. Furthermore, there was no evidence of sickness amongst local animals.

It was eight days after her return that she was taken ill. On this point alone it is just possible that she contracted plague whilst on holiday for the incubation period is two to eight days. So far as could be ascertained the origin of the child's illness remained unexplained. There was no connection with any sick person in the district nor was there any evidence of illness in the vicinity. Subsequent information about the wildlife in the area put a different complexion on things, however, especially since two or three dead hares had been found in a neighbouring field and a dead cat upon the doorstep of an immediately adjoining cottage two days before the child's illness. It is possible that the child had had contact with the sick cat or even the dead hares from which fleas could have been acquired.

The evidence suggests that the child may have become infected from a wild animal but that subsequent cases were caused by direct personal infection. All four cases were diagnosed as having pneumonia but the evidence in the first case suggested that this was a secondary and not a primary phenomenon. This conclusion supports the view that the infection had been acquired from a flea bite. The report summarises the cases by pointing out that the pneumonia which is associated with plague is usually a lobular and not a lobar pneumonia, and consequently the lungs do not present either on percussion or auscultation the characteristic signs of lobar pneumonia. One of the characteristic features of pneumonic plague is that the general condition of the patient is much more serious than the physical condition of the lungs would seem to warrant. In this series of cases the several medical men who saw and examined them were puzzled as to their nature, and it was the anomalous character of the symptoms and physical signs which led to a bacteriological examination being made.

TABLE 11

Sites of mortality amongst rats and hares in Suffolk

Year	Species	Locality	Distance from Freston outbreak
1906–7	Brown rat	Woolverstone Park	1½ miles N.E.
1906–7 & Autumn 1910	Brown rat	Shotley	5 miles E.S.E.
1906–7 & Autumn 1910	Brown rat	Erwarton	4 miles S.E.
1906–7 & Autumn 1910	Brown rat	Chelmondiston	2½ miles E.S.E.
1906–7 & Autumn 1910	Brown rat	Harkstead	2½ miles S.S.E.
1906–7	Hare	Woolverstone Park	1½ miles N.E.
1906–7	Rabbit	Woolverstone Park	1½ miles N.E.

There was evidence of mortality amongst rats and hares at several sites in Suffolk (Table 11) and in all cases the evidence from landowners and gamekeepers pointed to a heavy mortality, apparently from natural causes. In those days a rodenticide named 'Liverpool Virus' was widely used: this was a preparation of *Salmonella* sp.[13] and one of its effects on the rodents it killed was to cause severe wasting. Despite the fact that Liverpool Virus had been used on the Woolverstone Park estate in April 1910 there was no evidence of wasting in any of the dead animals. Even using poison it is rare to find many dead rats in the countryside and under normal circumstances dead rats are not found. As an animal which is preyed upon by a large number of natural predators, few rats live long enough to die of old age. The one circumstance under which rats and other rodents die in the field and are found in numbers is when there is an epizootic of plague in the rodent population.

Evidence and extent of plague amongst rodents

On 8 October 1910 a dead rat from Freston Wood (G on Fig. 11) was sent for examination along with a hare found dead at a point one mile south of the outbreak (H). Later in the month a cat found dead at Stutton Rectory (2¼ miles south west of Freston) and a ferret and rat from Freston were also examined. On bacteriological evidence it was believed that these animals had died of plague.

Rats and hares were collected from many sites in Suffolk, Essex and

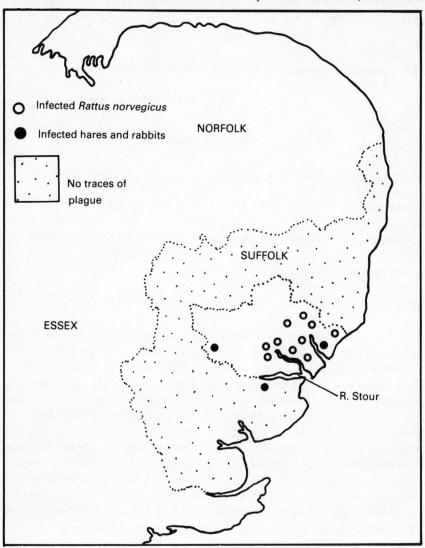

Fig. 12 The extent of plague in rats, hares and rabbits in East Anglia

Cambridgeshire. This revealed that plague in rats and hares extended well beyond the almost peninsula-like Samford Rural District and existed 15 miles to the west, 12 miles to the north-east and south of the River Stour (see Fig. 12).

Before going on to analyse the origin and spread of plague in this area it is as well to draw attention to other probable outbreaks of human plague which occurred a few miles away. These took place in the winters of 1906–7 and 1909–10 and the Freston outbreak drew public attention to them. Full data were not available but much time was spent collecting evidence and despite some gaps in the account it appears that both these outbreaks were very similar to the one at Freston.

The Trimley outbreak

At a point marked (C) on Figure 11 an outbreak occurred in a cottage whose seven occupants were in poor circumstances. The first attack began on 19 December 1909 and between then and the recovery of the last case in late January 1910, four people died and three became ill but recovered. As at Freston the course of the disease from onset to death was swift, in two cases as little as two days. In this outbreak there was considerable swelling at the angle of the jaw and in the groin, these enlargements being presumably lymph nodes.

The medical men who were in contact with these cases admitted that they had not seen anything like this before and they were unable to classify the illness. All the facts pointed to the presence of a communicable, highly fatal disease with a short incubation period. The occurrence of a secondary case at Nacton (D on Fig. 11) raises certain questions. During the illness in the household, two of the children, boys aged 12 and six, were removed to Barham Workhouse near Claydon on 11 January. On 16 January a daughter aged 19 went to visit her sick brother but due to an accident to her horse she was unable to return home and was taken in by a householder at Nacton (D). There she was taken ill on 19 January and on 23 January was removed to hospital where she eventually recovered. In the household where she had stayed a child of seven was taken ill on 3 February and died on 6 February. Before this child died her deteriorating condition had indicated the need for an exploratory operation and this was carried out. The surgeon reported that the omentum and mesentery were full of enlarged glands varying in size from a pea to a marble. In the light of subsequent events he was strongly of the opinion that the child was suffering from plague.

The author of the report considered that the short incubation period, together with the buboes, suggested plague rather than any other disease, and whilst influenza and typhus fever could be considered on the grounds of infectivity, the presence of buboes made it likely that the Trimley cases were those of either bubonic or septicaemic plague.

The Nacton case is not easy to explain. There are two possibilities: that it was of separate origin or was a secondary case arising from contact with the girl who stayed there before becoming ill.

The 19-year-old girl who recovered returned to Nacton on 2 February and the following day the girl of seven became ill. If she became infected from the recovering 19-year-old the incubation period was short, below the average incubation period of plague, although the Report of the Indian Plague Commission furnishes instances of periods of eight hours and 24 hours. If, on the other hand, the small child was infected before the elder left for hospital on 22 January when she was ill, this would mean an incubation period of 12 days. Unless the disease had taken the form of *pestis minor* and then, when the patient's resistance fell, developed into typical plague, this period would be too long.

Rats had been found dead of plague in Trimley parish in the autumn of 1910 and may have been present at the time of the outbreak.

The Shotley outbreak

The Freston outbreak attracted attention to an outbreak of fatal and infectious pneumonia which had occurred at Shotley (E and F on map) in December 1906 and January 1907. Eight people were taken ill and six died. Pneumonia was evident in these cases and the time between onset and death was short, usually about three days. Although influenza was present in the area at the time the rapidly fatal nature of the outbreak suggests that it more closely resembled pneumonic plague than influenza.

Plague in rats and lagomorphs in East Suffolk in November and December 1910

During this period it was shown that rats were infected with plague over a large area between Ipswich and the east coast. In addition, two hares were shown to have died of the disease and two rabbits were infected with plague (Fig. 12). A total of 719 rats (*Rattus norvegicus*) was examined, 568 in November and 151 in December.

The investigators carried out a survey of the ectoparasites (fleas only) on the rats and, since this is a very important factor in plague transmission, the details are of interest. Fleas from the rats at the time of examination were recorded and in addition those from six rats' nests which were dug out of banks. Three were from Suffolk, two from Elstree in Hertfordshire and one from Romsey in Hampshire.

Flea species on the rats
The fleas found in the nests were obtained in December. The Romsey nest was at the bottom of some hay in a barn but the others were found in ground

burrows and all nests were occupied by rats at the time they were found.

In this survey the flea *Xenopsylla cheopis* was not found. This species is the one commonly found in rat plague outbreaks and may be the predominant species present. At the beginning of this century in the Punjab and in Bombay *X. cheopis* was the common rat flea, 98 per cent of the fleas found on *Rattus rattus* belonging to this species (Plague Research Commission, 1907). This flea constituted 80–90 per cent of rat fleas in Sydney and Brisbane and 42 fleas from 150 rats (*Rattus norvegicus* and *Rattus rattus*) in Manila were all *X. cheopis*. Tiraboschi (1903–4; 1906–7) found that the same species was common on rats in Italy, at Caserta, Treviso and Genoa, being especially common in the last place where it formed 40 per cent of the fleas on ship rats. It formed a large proportion of the fleas from rats in San Francisco and made up 25 per cent of the flea population on ship rats in Marseilles.

Commenting upon the distribution of *Xenopsylla cheopis*, Rothschild (1906) said that the opinion he had formed with regard to the different species of fleas found on house and port rats all over the world was that, except in northern and central Europe, *Pulex cheopis* (= *X. cheopis*) was the commonest rat flea and in some localities was almost the only flea found upon rats. The extreme rarity of this species of flea in northern Europe and the fact that it is one of the commonest fleas found on rats in warm climates is perhaps a very important factor in an assessment of bubonic plague in Britain.

The Suffolk researchers did not find upon the rats they examined any specimens of *Pulex irritans*, the human flea, or *Ctenopsylla musculi*, the mouse flea. The latter was recorded at that time as being very common on rats from several places. It was claimed to be the most common parasite on *Rattus rattus* in Italy (Tiraboschi, 1906–7). It was the common rat flea in St Petersburg (Verjbitski, 1908) and out of 250 fleas from ships in Marseilles, 178 were *Ct. musculi*. Twenty-five per cent of the fleas from rats in Sydney in 1909 were of this species and according to Rothschild (1906) it was common on the house mouse in Great Britain and Northern Ireland and was sometimes present in considerable quantity on rats.

The Suffolk team did not find *Ctenocephalus felis*, the cat flea, nor *Ct. canis*, the dog flea. They did, however, find the species *Ceratophyllus fasciatus*, said to be commonly found on *Rattus norvegicus* in Europe and occurring elsewhere as well (Rothschild, 1910). This author (1906) said that although *Rattus rattus* was rare in the British Isles, on the few occasions when its fleas had been examined they had been *C. fasciatus*. This same flea was occasionally found on the house mouse, *Mus musculus*.

The other flea species found was *Ctenopthalmus agyrtes*. Rothschild (1910) said that this flea was common in England on field-mice and bank voles and occurred also on *Rattus norvegicus* when captured in the open. The Suffolk enquiry showed that it was a usual parasite of the rat and made up more than half of the total of 1,065 fleas from rats and their nests in East Suffolk, Elstree and Romsey. This flea may easily be mistaken for *Ctenopsylla musculi* and it is possible that reports of *Ct. musculi* on rats may in fact refer to *Ct. agyrtes*.

Flea species on the rabbits
Of 115 fleas recovered from 40 rabbits, 113 were *Spinopsyllus cuniculi*, the rabbit flea, and two were *Ceratophyllus fasciatus*. Since two rabbits infected with plague were found in the same locality, this finding is of some importance.

Feeding on man
Experiments showed that *Ceratophyllus fasciatus* fed readily on man. *Ctenopthalmus agyrtes*, however, seemed to rarely bite man. The rabbit flea, *Sp. cuniculi*, fed on man.

Flea prevalence
The prevalence of fleas is important in determining the outbreak of the rat epizootic and the subsequent spread of the disease to man. This fact was emphasised by the Commission for the Investigation of the Plague in India and flea infestation was the only factor that could be correlated with plague outbreaks. The epidemic season in widely differing parts of India with different climates in every case occurred during some portion of that period of the year in which there was an increase in flea prevalence. This could increase as much as six times.

In Suffolk the number of fleas per rat varied from 0.1 to 3.3 but was on average one flea per rat. It is significant that the greatest number of fleas was taken from samples of rats from districts which showed the highest proportion of plague-infected animals.

Despite this the number of fleas per rat was low. The Plague Research Commission present figures showing a higher infestation level: in the Punjab the number of *X. cheopis*, depending on the time of year, varied from two to 12.6 per rat. In Bombay the figure was two to seven, in Belgaum from 3.6 to 18.6 and in Poona from one to 11, with an average of 5.7 per rat in July and 9.1 per rat in August 1908.

Furthermore, as 50 per cent of the Suffolk rat fleas were *Ctenopthalmus agyrtes* which showed little inclination to bite man, this reduced the effective flea prevalence to about 0.5 fleas per rat. In India this level of infestation was insufficient to give rise to a human epidemic despite the greater contact between man and rat fleas. The Suffolk observations were made in November when flea breeding had probably ceased and it is possible that during the warmer weather a higher index would have been seen. Even today there are few data on rat flea numbers in Britain so that there is no means of knowing what seasonal variation exists and what summer flea levels can be expected.

Fleas infected with Y. pestis
The stomach contents of three fleas from a rat infected with plague were

examined and two of them contained large numbers of bacilli microscopically indistinguishable from plague bacilli.

Number of infected rats

Between 8 November 1910 and 2 January 1911, 719 live rats were captured and of these 20 were infected with plague. At the three sites from which most of the infected rats were recovered, 11 per cent were infected (14 out of 122). At the height of the epizootic in Bombay the infection rate only once reached six per cent so that although the total number examined in Suffolk was small there is every indication that a severe epizootic existed. At another site a heavy rat mortality had taken place two to four weeks earlier and a gamekeeper had found between 200 and 300 dead rats. In one site near marshes he collected 49 and from the same bank the investigators dug out a burrow containing 12 dead rats. Ten were too far decayed to allow diagnosis but two less-decomposed rats proved to be plague-infected.

Plague amongst rabbits

Two out of 40 rabbits had plague and organisms recovered from them killed rabbits, guinea-pigs and rats, all of whom presented a pathology characteristic of plague and from whose organs pure cultures of *Y. pestis* were obtained.

Observations on the Suffolk outbreak

The extent of the area in which plague-infected wild animals were recovered was considerable, approximately 207 square miles. This was a most substantial bridgehead and it is remarkable, despite apparently severe epizootics amongst the rodent population, that plague had not manifested itself more often in the human population before the Freston outbreak. The foothold which plague makes in any new area and from which, given the right conditions, it will extend into the surrounding countryside or town, appeared to have long since passed in Suffolk with such a widespread area of infection in evidence. In recent times where plague has entered a new region via a port the time elapsing before the disease has spread into the surrounding area has been considerable due to the difficulty of murine plague entering the sylvatic phase in the endemic rodent species, as in South Africa at the beginning of this century.

The source of plague in Suffolk was never determined although the assumption that plague-infected rats were off-loaded with excess grain at Butterman's Bay in order to lighten ships proceeding to Ipswich seems reasonable. That point is, moreover, near the centre of the area in which infected animals were caught. From here it is 18 miles to the most distant plague-infected animal. If rodent mortality back in 1906–7 was due to epizootics of plague, as it appeared to be in 1910–11, then, even assuming that plague entered the area in 1906 and had spread outwards during the four years following, it would only represent a spread of roughly four miles per year. This could be a maximum figure, for the high mortality in 1906–7 at several places indicates that plague must have been introduced even earlier and this would reduce the figure to less than four miles per year.

Quite independently of the details contained in the official report I have obtained interesting information on rats from an estate at Elveden in West Suffolk between Thetford and Mildenhall. This was an area in which rats trapped in the survey were shown to be plague-free. Estate records of Brown rats killed annually show peak years in 1907 and 1910 and earlier in both 1903 and 1904. Without knowing the nature of the trapping pressure and the area involved, it is impossible to make truly valid comparisons between years but it is likely that these were similar in the years preceding World War I, the reduction in gamekeepers and the changes in land usage not being apparent until during and after the war. Nevertheless, it is temping to consider that the epizootic might have extended over a much larger area than was thought by the enquiry, the absence of human cases failing to draw attention to it.

Epizootics coupled with rodent control presumably eradicated plague from the area for there has been no repetition of these events in the British Isles. Despite the fact that *Rattus norvegicus* was widely distributed throughout the area, an almost entirely agricultural one, there does not appear to have been any evidence that plague became sylvatic in, for example, field-mice. The Suffolk enquiry showed that the rat carried large numbers of *Ctenopthalmus agyrtes*, a flea said by Rothschild to be the usual one found on the field-mouse. If plague had transferred to the mice and even produced epizootics it is unlikely that the deaths of field-mice would have been noticed and the simple experiments carried out showed that *Ct. agyrtes* was reluctant to bite man. However, I am inclined to believe that plague never entered the sylvatic phase in Suffolk for this reason: assuming a transfer to field-mice, the most ubiquitous British mammal, with a flea shared by rats, then a return transfer from mice to rats was a real possibility on various occasions and this would have led to rat epizootics which must have been noticed. If plague did not leave the widely scattered rural Brown rats and enter the endemic mammalian species in 1906–11 when rat and field-mouse contact must have been close, then it is not surprising that there was no resultant sylvatic plague from the plague of 1348 when, supposing it was plague, it would have been carried by *Rattus rattus*, a species more closely confined to human habitations in the British climate.

The Suffolk enquiry spent some time considering the differences between conditions in East Suffolk and those in India from the point of view of their epidemiological importance. Drawing on the experience of the then recent Plague Research Commission they expressed the conclusions thus:

> (1) in the majority of cases, during an epidemic of plague, man contracts the disease from plague-infected rats through the agency of plague-infected rat fleas;

(2) the chance of human infection is determined by the number of hungry infected rat fleas, provided they will feed on man, and his accessibility for them.

So far as conditions went in Suffolk, certain points are clear. Rat plague existed and rats which died of plague had a septicaemia comparable to that seen in India. At least half of the fleas on the rats belonged to a species which readily bit man and there were plague bacilli in the stomachs of fleas from infected rats. There was no reason to suppose that such fleas could not transmit plague, yet there had been very few cases. The epizootic severity in certain parts of Suffolk would, in India, have spread the disease to man.

The number of fleas in Suffolk was smaller than in India and little more can be said on that score. The authors considered that the main difference between India and Suffolk was in regard to the accessibility of man for rat fleas. In India *Rattus rattus* is a highly domesticated animal and literally shares living space with people, rats and nests being among the household possessions, especially in peasants' single rooms which serve all purposes. In such a room the Commission found 263 rat fleas.

Rattus norvegicus, on the other hand, is not allowed to have the same close contact since Europeans, unlike Indians, destroy rats. The Brown rat therefore lives mainly outside dwellings and in summer, when fleas are most abundant, probably moves further from habitations to live in hedgerows.

On the question of the flea species involved, Hirst (1953) has pointed out that whilst *Nosopsyllus* (= *Ceratophyllus*) *fasciatus* can transmit plague from one rodent to another in the laboratory it does not do it so well as *Xenopsylla cheopis* and even if it were as efficient as the latter it would be bound to play a subordinate role in the field on account of its inability to breed apart from the nest of its host. He considers it to be probably more important as a reservoir of plague infection in the rat burrow than as an active transmitter of disease rat to man or colony to colony of rats and thus plays a relatively insignificant part in the production of major epizootics or epidemics, 'in so far as is known plague epidemics have never occurred in communities where *fasciatus* existed alone and were not associated with *cheopis*. The role of *N. fasciatus*, then, is to prolong an enzootic initiated by *X. cheopis*, such an enzootic being seldom reflected in significant human mortality'. He cites the Seattle enzootic which smouldered for ten years with only three human cases and the British outbreaks in Glasgow, Liverpool, Cardiff, Hull, Bristol and London referred to earlier in this chapter in support of this. However, although *X. cheopis* was lacking in Suffolk, there was evidence of severe epizootic plague in the rats.

Hirst presumes that the *R. rattus* of London in past centuries had a high proportion of *N. fasciatus* but finds it difficult to believe that all, or nearly all, their fleas would have consisted of this species since there is no evidence anywhere today that *N. fasciatus* could have supported a severe rat epizootic in London without the assistance of a substantial proportion of *X. cheopis*. The question is: what proportion of *X. cheopis* would be required? The *cheopis* index, i.e. fleas per rat, of the Colombo endemic zone was 0.8–1.2 and between one and two in areas where plague was spreading in India and Ceylon.

Surveys of rat fleas in Britain have shown that on London rats the *N. fasciatus* index rose to 3.5 towards the end of the year, 80 per cent of the catch being of that species, most of the rest *Leptopsylla segnis* and only two *X. cheopis* on a *Rattus rattus* in the south-west India Dock. Hirst trapped 100 *Rattus norvegicus* at London Zoo in September 1937. All the fleas were *N. fasciatus* with an average of 3.8 per rat. Foci of *X. cheopis* have been present in London; for example, in 1911 this flea multiplied in a nest near warm pipes in the underground portion of Guy's Hospital, the host being *Rattus norvegicus*. Balfour (1922) said that in England *X. cheopis* was the only flea on 34 *Rattus rattus*, comprising 5.9 per cent of the ectoparasites, and on 444 *R. norvegicus* it was slightly more abundant than *Ceratophyllus fasciatus*, making up 3.6 per cent of the ectoparasites against 3.2 per cent for the latter flea.

Pointing out that *X. cheopis* existed in London and was able to breed even under the unfavourable conditions of today Hirst (1953) said, 'Undoubtedly it must have been far more abundant on the vast colonies of black rats which shared with man the warm dwelling rooms and kitchens of seventeenth century London'. However, the conditions of 'today', the early 1950s, were probably much better for the fleas than those of seventeenth-century London. Most buildings in London today are incomparably warmer and the indoor temperatures day and night vary less and are almost certainly more favourable for *X. cheopis*.

X. cheopis has been common in docks in some British ports. In Liverpool in 1921 it bred on rats all the year round with 4.3 fleas per rat, even in winter and in Plymouth in 1938, 2.8 fleas per rat were found on *R. norvegicus*. Between 1926 and 1928, 86 per cent of the rats of Cardiff ships and docks were *Rattus rattus*, 78 per cent of their fleas being *X. cheopis*. In the docks, 91 per cent of the rats were *Rattus rattus* and 28 per cent of fleas *X. cheopis*.

These two flea species are quite different in their temperature requirements. In all stages except the imaginal, temperatures below 7.2°C are fatal to *X. cheopis* whereas the eggs of *N. fasciatus* can hatch at an average temperature of 5°C and a temperature of 7.2°C is quite suitable for this hardy species. To enable *X. cheopis* to breed, a minimum temperature of around 15.5°C is necessary. Thus, unless *Rattus norvegicus* nested in warm situations, *X. cheopis* could not breed on it and out of doors this rat could not support many *X. cheopis* in the winter.

Hirst points out that the plague season in Old London, i.e. the seventeenth century, corresponds exactly with the period that would be expected if *X. cheopis* were the chief vector. That flea species in a temperate climate would reach a maximum density in the late summer and autumn, following a warm summer and requiring an average temperature of from 18.3°C–21.1°C for rapid increase. He states that three *X. cheopis* plus two *N. fasciatus* per rat would be enough to maintain the Great Plague of London. The ideal plague combination would therefore be *Rattus rattus*, an indoor rat, with *Xenopsylla cheopis*, an indoor flea. It is interesting that Hirst makes this important point, recognising that for plague to have been effective in the temperate latitudes this partnership would be necessary. The widespread nature of the Black Death with its severe effect on villages in a cold climatic period is difficult to reconcile with these biological essentials. Even if *Rattus norvegicus* had been present with *Nosopsyllus fasciatus* or *Leptopsylla segnis* as its main fleas, plague would not have been active because, as Hirst maintains, a territory infested with this combination of rat and flea must be far more resistant to plague infection than one harbouring *Rattus rattus* with *Xenopsylla cheopis*. He says, finally, 'East Anglia appears to be the only region so far discovered where field rodent plague has disappeared once it had become widespread in the woods and fields. It seems then that plague among both rural and urban colonies of *Rattus norvegicus* in England has a tendency to self extinction.'

In Suffolk, between 1910 and 1918, there was human plague (a further two plague deaths occurred not far from Shotley in June 1918) and probable human plague between 1906 and 1918 with a presumptive rat enzootic between 1906 and 1918. Pneumonic plague was present in most cases and therefore there was a focus of the disease in a form capable of rapid diffusion. As we have seen already, during the early part of this century the pneumonic form frequently occurred yet, despite being locally severe, as in Manchuria, never became a pandemic. Shrewsbury (1971) says that pneumonic plague cannot occur in the absence of the bubonic disease and cannot persist as an independent form of plague. The reason for this is because the effects of pneumonic plague are severe, the very high case mortality ensuring that few, if any, survive and hence such outbreaks are short lived. Thus, in the absence of a reservoir of infected rats the pneumonic form of plague cannot endure for very long.

The diffusibility of pneumonic plague shows a great deal of variation. General examples of the slow spread of this variant of the disease have already been given from both tropical and temperate latitudes and at this point it is worth looking in a little more detail at one of these and some further outbreaks. In those localities which suffered severely from bubonic plague during the early part of the current pandemic, e.g. India, Java and Hong Kong, the incidence of pneumonic plague has been low, one to five per cent (Petrie and Todd, 1923). Seal (1969) says that the incidence of pneumonic plague in India was generally below one per cent (of total plague cases) and never exceeded three per cent in any year since 1895. These are hard facts and although Wu, Lien-Teh (1926) says that the pneumonic form of plague was rather frequent in the early days of the present pandemic in India, he gives no details to support this comment. He further considers that the pneumonic form was often frequent in newly invaded areas, but inconspicuous later on in the same foci and that this seems to have been the course of the Black Death: the pneumonic type being rampant early in the pandemic but, wherever the plague persisted, it became less fatal. He is of the opinion that a similar evolution took place in later centuries when plague was re-imported into Europe.

It is curious that Wu, Lien-Teh should imply that pneumonic plague was so severe in the Black Death, because in his account of plague in the Orient (Wu, Lien-Teh, 1922) he goes to some pains to quote experiments and field experience which show a low infectivity for the pneumonic form. He describes how guinea-pigs and rabbits were placed in the sick rooms of patients suffering from pneumonic plague before and after their death and shows how few of these became infected. The same species were also placed in coffins containing clothes freshly removed from the dead and none of them died. He concluded from this that the sick room by itself, and even when occupied by plague patients, was not particularly dangerous except when standing in the direct line of the spit or droplet.

He goes on to quote cases where patients with fever and cough travelled in railway cars with 47, 37, 47 and 30 other persons for more than nine hours and yet, despite the close proximity of the pneumonic plague-infected person, none of these other passengers became ill.

An epidemic of bubonic plague in man is dependent upon an epizootic in the rats living in close proximity. As a rule, when the rat epizootic and the transfer of fleas ceases, the epidemic also comes to an end and although it is possible that pneumonic cases may arise and theoretically initiate a fresh epidemic by droplet transmission, this is rare and occurs only under exceptional conditions. It is worth remembering that the man to man infectivity of bubonic plague has also been exaggerated, as data from India show. Bannerman (1906) pointed out that during the plague in Bombay few, if any, attendants on plague patients in the hospitals were attacked and, when they were, some other cause was found apart from the patients they attended; for example in the plague hospital at the Old Government House at Parel there were 533 cases yet none of the attendants got plague and out of 140 attendants the only one to develop plague had assisted at post mortem examinations although it is not clear that this was the cause of his infection. Two hundred and forty friends attended the sick yet none of them became infected. At another hospital which treated 374 plague cases none of the staff were infected and neither were about 400 people visiting the sick or remaining at their bedside. Altogether in 28 hospitals there were 9,631 cases with 764 attendants. Of these, 36 became cases but only 12 were infected in the hospitals and another eight had attended pneumonic cases and became infected.

In Bombay hospitals in 1898–9, of the total number of cases, 5.8 per cent were of primary plague pneumonia and a further 3.6 per cent were cases of secondary pneumonia. Thus, almost 9.5 per cent of cases were potentially dangerous from the point of view of direct man to man infection. The fact that a pneumonic plague epidemic did not result was doubtless because primary pneumonic plague epidemics rarely, if ever, occur in the absence of constantly low temperatures and high relative humidity. A few severe epidemics of plague have been of the primary pneumonic type transmitted man to man by droplet infection from the cough but the spread or failure to spread is due to weather conditions. Freezing temperatures with a high relative humidity favour transmission since pulverised and frozen sputum and cough droplets retain virulent bacilli and hence infection for a long time. In those communities where there is overcrowding and close contact between the sick and the fit and where insanitary conditions and practices are normal this form of plague thrives. The immediate origin of such outbreaks is usually isolated cases of secondary plague pneumonia occurring as a complication during bubonic or primary septicaemic plague. Blount (1976) says that such secondary pneumonia is not as infectious as is primary pneumonic plague, and unless the conditions for respiratory transmission are totally suitable it is less apt to initiate large epidemics. In the light of this information it is unlikely that pneumonic plague could have been responsible for extensive epidemics in the British Isles because the necessary climatic conditions would rarely be right. Even if winter temperatures were low the relative humidity would only be favourable in fuggy, crowded buildings and it is very likely that medieval buildings in the British Isles were usually cold. The evidence is not convincing that the pneumonic form was prevalent early in the Black Death for although it is true that pulmonary symptoms were evident, so also were the other manifestations and as we shall see later most of these could have resulted from organisms other than plague bacillus. There is no real evidence that the pneumonic form became less fatal as plague persisted in the pandemic.

If we can accept that bubonic plague was not biologically feasible then this reduces the claims for a pneumonic plague epidemic which arises as a secondary manifestation of bubonic plague (Wu, Lien-Teh, 1922). Furthermore, it would be unlikely that the pneumonic form would have been active at all the times of year that the 1348–9 epidemic was. The rapid rate of diffusion favours a droplet-borne respiratory disease or a highly contagious disease rather than one depending upon two vectors and such a hypothesis could better account for the spread across sparsely populated areas of the country.

Christopher Morris (1971), in a detailed review of Shrewsbury's exhaustive history of bubonic plague in Britain, takes him to task for ignoring the evidence in favour of a high percentage of pneumonic cases in the Great Pestilence of 1348–50. It is quite clear that there were many cases in England and elsewhere which indicated a pulmonary involvement but it is quite another matter to be certain that they were specifically pneumonic plague. Morris suggests that Shrewsbury's myopia concerning pneumonic plague arose from the latter's statement that 'pneumonic plague cannot occur in the absence of the bubonic form and it cannot persist as an independent form of plague'. Morris points to the great pneumonic epidemics of 1910–11 and 1920–1 (the first having been elsewhere referred to by Shrewsbury (1964) as exclusively pneumonic plague disseminated by human contacts) as evidence that this is not the case.

Shrewsbury says that the Manchurian epidemic of plague in 1910–11 had its origin in an epizootic of the disease among the marmots which at that time were in demand in the fur trade. Many of the hunters were Chinese with little experience and they became infected because of their inexperience in handling diseased animals. In them the disease became pneumonic and was greatly aided as a result of the extreme cold of the Manchurian winter and the severe overcrowding in the small townships where the hunters congregated. He concludes, 'The resulting epidemic was exclusively one of pneumonic plague and was disseminated solely by human contacts'. Shrewsbury is only accurate in his remark that pneumonic plague cannot *persist* as an independent form of plague in the sense that whilst it will on rare occasions be present as a severe epidemic, this will end either when climatic conditions cease to favour its dissemination or because the rapid and high mortality ensures few survivors and the outbreak comes to an abrupt end. Pneumonic plague cannot persist in enzootic form and this is probably what Shrewsbury had in mind.

As Wu, Lien-Teh *et al.* (1936) have pointed out, a fundamental difference between bubonic and pneumonic epidemics lies in their individual relations to epizootics:

> a bubonic epidemic is dependent upon infection among rodents both for its origin and throughout its course. Pneumonic epidemics are usually not of direct rodent origin, human cases with secondary pneumonia intervening. Once primary pneumonic develops it takes its course independent of the epizootics, the infection being conveyed from man to man. Frequently, in a locality invaded by pneumonic plague, epizootics are totally absent, infection having been imported from another place by patients.

However, murine plague rarely seems to give rise to severe primary pneumonic outbreaks. It is important to remember that pneumonic plague basically cannot occur without the existence of plague in a rodent population and it is the existence of such a population which is fundamental to the disease in any form at all. Wu, Lien-Teh *et al.* (1936) in a discussion of the origins of pneumonic cases emphasise the point that primary pneumonic plague is usually traceable to bubonic cases with well-marked secondary lung involvement. Implicit in this is the presence of infected rodents and fleas. Furthermore, although Shrewsbury has omitted Wu, Lien-Teh's treatise on pneumonic plague from his bibliography (Wu, Lien-Teh, 1926), it is worth pointing out that in all fairness to Shrewsbury's remarks, Wu, Lien-Teh (1922) in his paper on the Manchurian outbreaks said, 'pneumonic plague epidemics arise as a secondary manifestation of bubonic plague'.

The Manchurian epidemics (Wu, Lien-Teh *et al.*, 1936) deserve a closer inspection because they are frequently quoted as examples of the fearful spreading capability of pneumonic plague should it arise in the world today. Yet the spread was due to certain extraordinary conditions, none of which were present in medieval Britain, and the death toll, considering the distance covered, was very small.

The first epidemic in 1910–11 was probably due indirectly to the great increase in the price of marmot skins which rose from 0.30 rouble in 1907 to 1.20 roubles in 1910. The exports of these skins increased from 700,000 in 1907 to 2,500,000 in 1910. This enormous increase was produced by an increase in the number of hunters: in the summer of 1910 there were 11,000 Chinese hunters at Manchouli and by October there were still 4,600 present.

Rodents dying of plague appear sick and drowsy and are easy prey. The native hunters were skilled and because they shot animals had learned to avoid sick marmots. The influx of get-rich-quick hunters consisted of unskilled Chinese who used snares and since these are unselective in catching animals the hunters had to handle sick animals and as a result became infected from them.

Despite being pneumonic (although there is little guarantee that every single early case was so) the evolution of the epidemic was slow and cases among the hunters occurred as early as April 1910 and continued throughout the summer. Although officially recorded at Manchouli, the hunters' centre, on 12 October, it was present a month before that date. This was too late to prevent the spread of the disease along the railway system, West to Siberia and East into China. Eastwards it spread to Tsitsikar and then to Mergen (halfway between Tsitsikar and Taheiho (Aigun) on the Amur). Harbin became the central focus of the epidemic which then spread to Hantaohotzu near the eastern border of Manchuria. It spread widely to the south: to Shuangchengpu, Changchun, Kirin, Mukden, Shanhaikwan, Dairen, Tientsin, Peking, Tsinan and Chefoo.

From Manchouli to Tsinan (Shantung) the disease covered 1700 miles during the period September to April and almost 60,000 people died. The epidemic spread directly along the railways so that in the course of a day infection might be carried scores of miles to a new focus.

Ten years later a second epidemic began and, although on this occasion the amount of hunting was not large, abnormal conditions were present in Transbaikalia, where there was civil war, and at the Manchurian stations which were overcrowded with retiring troops which made sanitary control difficult. The first cases occurred in the Chinese (formerly Mongolian) territory at Hailar, which was second only to Manchouli as a centre of the fur trade, during October and November. These early cases were at first *bubonic* in nature (Wu, Lien-Teh et al., 1936), but the later course of the epidemic was pneumonic.

In this outbreak unruly soldiers caused trouble and stopped all plague-preventive measures for one week, thereby allowing the disease to spread.

Two contacts set free by soldiers reached the coal mines at Dalainor, 100 miles west, and infected others in the crowded underground dwellings and it was this which began the epidemic. In this district, more than 1000 out of 4000 miners died. From Dalainor, persons who were incubating the disease fled 20 miles west to Manchouli where they caused the deaths of 1141. Others reached Tsitsikar where 1734 died and then Harbin where a further 3125 died. Once again Harbin was the centre of infection due to opposition from soldiers coupled with an ignorant populace. A few local outbreaks were contained and the disease was held south of Harbin; for example, there were only 77 deaths at Changchun compared with 5000 in 1911. From Harbin the plague went east in mid-February along the railway to Vladivostok where the first case was seen on 9 April. In this town the epidemic lasted all summer, ending in October with a total of 498 dead.

In this 1920–1 epidemic 9300 people died, the low death rate being due mainly to the efforts of Dr Lien-Teh Wu and his team in containing contacts so far as they were able. They said that, unlike the first epidemic, they never lost control of the second one.

Severe though these two outbreaks were, particularly the first, considering the great areas covered and the sizes of the towns involved the death toll was astonishingly low. Wu, Lien-Teh (1926) considered the infectivity of pneumonic plague amongst hospital staff and the general public and in the case of the former came to the conclusion that the hospital personnel had few infections because they were less exposed in hygienic wards than in poor hospitals and the hovels of patients. In the 1910–11 Manchurian epidemic one out of 60 deaths occurred among staff and these included burial and auxiliary personnel. In 1920–21 the proportion of staff in total cases was one in 129.

Concerning the general incidence of pneumonic plague, Wu, Lien-Teh (1926) considered that whilst this form of the disease had a great spreading power in cold weather, the infectivity of patients was not so absolute as some authors seemed to believe. Further, he said, 'In Manchuria, as in other plague areas, a short, close contact is often insufficient to produce infection. Likewise, the number of victims among the persons isolated after having been found in contact with plague patients is, as a rule, very low.' At Harbin in 1920–1 only eight per cent of contacts developed plague due to good detection in the isolation wagons and getting patients to hospital, but even at Dalainor, where discipline among miners could not be maintained, the incidence of cases did not exceed 21.9 per cent.

Upper Egypt, especially the southern provinces of Qena and Girga, showed a repeated tendency to become foci of pneumonic plague. Between 1899 and 1913 there were 88 pure outbreaks of pneumonic plague in Egypt. Table 12 shows the details of nine pure pneumonic plague outbreaks, each of which had over 30 cases, in Egypt from 1906 to 1912. The percentage of the population infected is low, the highest being 1.69 per cent at El Hamidat. This was true of the whole 88 outbreaks, the majority of them remaining isolated.

TABLE 12

Number of cases of pneumonic plague expressed as a percentage of total population in 9 outbreaks of pure pneumonic plague in Egypt, 1906–12

Town or village	Year	Population	Number of cases	Duration of outbreak	% of total population
Dishna	1906	10,386	143	Mar.June	1.38
Isna	1907	19,103	73	Mar. 21–May 27	0.38
Dishna	1907	10,386	36	Feb. 16–May 7	0.35
El Makhadma	1907	7,067	33	Apr. 9–May 6	0.47
Karnak	1908	12,585	78	Apr. 10–May 20	0.62
Maragha	1908	8,789	32	Feb. 4–29	0.36
Waburat Armant	1910	5,780	41	Apr. 17–May 21	0.71
El Hamidat	1911	3,728	63	Feb. 27–Mar. 18	1.69
Edfa	1912	6,662	45	Jun. 6–July 3	0.68

Occasionally, contacts escaped from the primary outbreak and introduced the disease into neighbouring villages, yet there were seldom more than three or four secondary offshoots. Thus, although foci were apt to flare up in affected districts, the outbreaks that followed were characterised by low diffusibility. It must, however, be added that the Egyptian medical authorities were aware of the potential dangers of pneumonic plague spreading and took quick action to prevent suspects leaving and to isolate the sick whenever possible so that it is not a strictly direct comparison with the Middle Ages where total ignorance prevailed. Nevertheless, the spread of pneumonic plague was less rapid than is generally thought and modern evidence scarcely bears out the belief that the extremely swift passage of medieval plague can be explained on the grounds that the pneumonic form was prevalent, especially since many communities were isolated and shunned if there was any hint of disease.

In Egypt the family incidence was the most distinctive feature of the outbreaks: the occurrence of several deaths in a family being in itself highly suggestive of pneumonic plague. For example, in Edfa village in June 1912, out of a total of 45 cases, 40 were in one family group in ten houses in the village of 6662 inhabitants. Seal (1969) comments that outbreaks of primary pneumonic plague in India have usually been confined to a single or a few families only.

Because the most favourable conditions for the spread of pneumonic plague are those with a low temperature and high relative humidity, it is often assumed that this form of plague is absent in tropical and semi-tropical countries. However, apart from Egypt, the disease has arisen in other tropical areas. In 1908 plague was confirmed in the port of Accra, West Africa, most of the 168 cases being bubonic. It spread to outlying villages where the majority of 134 cases were pneumonic. In 1912 in an outbreak at Kilimanjaro 66 out of the 69 deaths which occurred were caused by pneumonic plague. The highest death rate recorded in Africa was in the village of Yoff, 15 kilometres from Dakar, where nearly 80 per cent of the population died (Lafont, 1915). In this outbreak *Mus musculus* (the house mouse) and *Rattus rattus* were the species involved in the murine epizootic.

In this century we have had the opportunity to study plague outbreaks in areas where the disease had never occurred before and whilst pneumonic plague was present it is misleading to state that it was frequent at first and later inconspicuous. In South Africa (Chapter 8) eighty per cent of the 766 cases in the epidemic of 1901 were bubonic. Of course, in most places where known plague arrived for the first time the new knowledge about the causation of the disease enabled the authorities to reduce cases over the years so that there has not been the opportunity to watch a natural spread in the human population comparable with that in medieval times.

Much of this chapter has been concerned with the apparent failure of plague to become established in the British Isles despite several introductions into large ports and a rural bridgehead in Suffolk in the early years of the twentieth century. It is an important aspect of true plague that its perpetuation in any newly colonised region will be largely dependent upon its transfer to the sylvatic state. It must be acknowledged that one of the curious aspects of alleged medieval plague in northern Europe has been its failure to become sylvatic despite a period of exposure of almost 400 years and this fact alone must give us food for thought when we compare this with plague on the other continents. In the British Isles not only plague but some other zoonotic diseases have failed to become established despite introductions which have in some cases been accurately documented. Rabies, which was formerly present in dogs, was eradicated towards the end of the nineteenth century, reintroduced in dogs over several counties after World War I yet despite this has failed to become established in the wild carnivore population. Leptospirosis, a serious disease carried by rodents, including rats, and infecting man and farm animals, shows a reduction in types across northern Europe from south-east to north-west, finally becoming almost non-existent in the islands to the west and north of Britain and in Ireland. I have elsewhere suggested (Twigg, 1980) that the islands comprising Great Britain, 'provide conditions which have not favoured the establishment of some important micro-organisms and appear to represent the end of a geographical line of success. The term "pathocline"[14] would not be inappropriate in representing the position of these and other parasitic organisms in the mammals of Britain and Western Europe'.

If there had been a widespread rural Black rat population in which plague alternated between an enzootic and an epizootic state it is most likely, from evidence elsewhere, that the disease would have entered the sylvatic state in one of the several available rodent species of the countryside. That there is no trace of *Yersinia pestis* in either British or north European field mammals I regard as good evidence against its original widespread position. It has been said that the absence of *Yersinia pestis* from endemic rodent species could be due to the fact that the bacterium has undergone mutation into *Yersinia pseudotuberculosis*, which does occur in the British Isles. However, there is no evidence that such genetic drift has occurred. Furthermore, if divergence such as this had taken place then, with the rapid generation time of bacteria and from known cases, it could just as easily have returned to *Yersinia pestis*. If divergence can be postulated, then with no less accuracy so can convergence.

It may be suggested that the plague bacillus of the fourteenth century possessed a greater virulence than that of the late nineteenth and early twentieth centuries and that this accounted for its enhanced performance. However, *Yersinia pestis* appears to be a stable organism without proliferation into the many serotypes that we see, for example, in leptospires or the many types of influenza. This would indicate that its character is unlikely to have changed to any marked degree over long periods of time.

It is important to remember that when the disease enters man it has almost entirely reached a biological dead end. Its continuation is only guaranteeed in rodents and it is to them that any degree of accommodation has to be made. The biology of both rodents and fleas is the key to plague perpetuation and the essential feature of my argument is that the effect of the plague bacillus in any new locality will be enhanced or diminished according to the environment and its ability to house suitable vectors, to the climatic factors influencing them, the density of people and rodents and the nature of the contact between the two, as well as to such things as transport, dwellings, agriculture and probably others too.

CHAPTER TEN

The pattern and effects
of a plague epidemic

Modern plague epidemiology may be said to date from the discovery of *B. pestis* by Yersin and Kitasato in 1894 (Plague Research Commission, 1907) and although it had long been known that there was a relationship between rat deaths and the human epidemic and that this formed the basis of rudimentary practical measures taken by primitive communities, it was not until 1897 that Yersin stated: 'Plague which is at first a disease of the rat soon becomes a disease of man'. By the turn of the century several research workers were engaged in determining the relation of rat plague to human outbreaks and many important observations were made.

The Indian Plague Commission (1901) summed up the evidence presented to them and considered that the chief importance of rats in the epidemiology of plague arose in connection with the first outbreak of the disease in an infected place. When plague was once established in a locality they believed human agency was a more important factor in spreading the disease than the agency of rats. This was an over-simplified and premature judgement, as later work was to show.

Various observations had led to the conclusion that general rat mortality went on increasing several weeks ahead of the human mortality. Studies in Hong Kong showed that the epidemic began a fortnight later than the epizootic, the climax of the epidemic being reached a fortnight later than that of the epizootic. In Mauritius the rat epizootic preceded the epidemic by two to four weeks; in some localities the epidemic did not cease till six to eight weeks after complete disappearance of the epizootic.

As the parts played by rats and fleas in plague dissemination came to be understood, the research workers in India carefully plotted the course of the epizootic and the corresponding epidemic and succeeded in quantifying the nature of the observed patterns. These models are therefore theoretically available to anyone wishing to compare known plague outbreaks, both bubonic and pneumonic, with the epidemics of past centuries. Of course, there is no record of the epizootic earlier than the current pandemic but the

(Each weekly figure is expressed as a percentage in terms of the mean of the year. Therefore all figures <100% go beneath the zero)

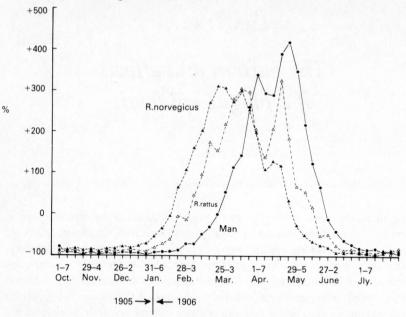

Fig. 13 Plague in *Rattus rattus*, *R. norvegicus* and man – Bombay city 1905–6 human mortality pattern is sometimes available.

Wu, Lien-Teh *et al.* (1936) stated a very important basic point concerning the curve of bubonic epidemics, the curve being the shape of the graph when the infection rates of rats or the number of human cases are plotted against time as in Figure 13. They pointed out that whenever infection of plague reached the rats of a hitherto plague-free region or when the disease became recrudescent after being carried over the off-season by a smouldering epizootic, the infection amount at first available would be limited. It was therefore to be expected that the rise of an epizootic and consequently that of the subsequent epidemic would necessarily be gradual. Others have emphasised the slow evolution of a bubonic plague epidemic and contrasted this with the explosive development of other epidemic diseases such as cholera. The second feature in the curve, pointed out by Wu, Lien-Teh *et al.* (1936) is that the decline after the peak is more abrupt than the rise because the factors which cut short an outbreak are more determinate than those which are responsible for its commencement. However, as we shall see later, the decline is not always more rapid than the rise, according to Brownlee (1918). The Plague Research Commission reached the general conclusions that the rise of an epizootic, and consequently of an epidemic, depended upon: (1) a suitable mean temperature below 29.4°C and above 10.0°C: a mean temperature around or below 10.0°C was likely to limit plague outbreaks by keeping down the number of plague-infected rats developing bacteraemia; (2) enough susceptible rats; and (3) enough rat fleas. Conversely, the decline of the epizootic and the epidemic was determined by some or all of the following: (1) a high mean temperature of 29.4°C or above: a plague epidemic was checked when the mean daily temperature went above 26.6°C and especially when it reached 29.4°C or 32.2°C, the adverse influence of such high temperatures being due to their action upon the infectivity of fleas; (2) a diminution in the total number of rats and an increase in the proportion of immune to susceptible animals; and (3) a diminution in the number of rat fleas.

If we now look at Figure 13 we can see the data for Bombay covering a period of 12 months, October 1905–September 1906 (Plague Research Commission, 1907a). Three curves are presented, one for human deaths and the other two for plague-infected *Rattus rattus* and *Rattus norvegicus*. It is clear that even in the 'off season' there were human cases and rat infection because at no time in any of the 52 weeks does any sample reach zero. The lowest number of human deaths in any one week, November 5–11, was six. Plague amongst the rats persisted during every month of the year in most sections of the city with *Rattus norvegicus* providing focal points of infection. As a result, when the various conditions favourable to flea breeding and bacilli multiplication began to improve, the effect was citywide. This is important because an epidemic in a large city which begins from the importation of one or two fleas or a rat at one point will develop in a quite different way, especially in so far as the time taken for the maximum development is concerned.

In Bombay we can see that the three curves are not all alike. The *Rattus norvegicus* line exhibits a peak in infection from 20 February–14 March, whereas the *Rattus rattus* curve has two peaks, the first one at around 14 March and the second around 17 April. After the peak the infection declines rapidly, especially in the case of *R. rattus*. The human curve also has two peaks, the first on 27 March and the second, main peak on 24 April. Again, as in the case of the rats the decline in deaths is rapid, unlike the more gradual increase of mortality before the peaks.

Clearly, the three peaks do not coincide with one another yet there is some similarity in shape between plague in *R. rattus* and in man, the peak in *R. norvegicus* being further removed from the human peaks than the first *R. rattus* peak. *Rattus rattus* appears to be more responsible for the human epidemic than does *Rattus norvegicus*, a fact which seems wholly reasonable in view of the proximity of the Black rat to man. The interval between the *R. rattus* epizootic and the human epidemic is between ten and 14 days, a period which can be divided into three parts: (a) the period elapsing between the death of a rat and the communication of infection from rat to man by the rat flea – three days; (b) the incubation period in man – a mean of three days; (c) the duration of illness in a fatal case – a mean of five and a half days. A mean figure of 11½ days for the interval between epizootic and epidemic fits the observed data well. In Bombay the *Rattus norvegicus* epizootic preceded the

Rattus rattus epizootic by a mean interval of about ten days, suggesting a train of events with similar timing between the two rat species.

The authors of the study of the epidemiological observations in Bombay (Plague Research Commission, 1907a) concluded that *Rattus norvegicus* was perhaps responsible for plague in *Rattus rattus* and, furthermore, because *norvegicus* was found more away from houses, in stables etc, and tended to range further afield, it would be chiefly responsible for the diffusion among the rats throughout the city. As we have seen, plague persisted during the off season, this persistence being due chiefly to *Rattus norvegicus*. If this is correct then it would mean that in fourteenth-century Britain, in the absence of *Rattus norvegicus*, plague would be very slow spreading in *Rattus rattus* since the cold climate would serve to localise that species even further.

Brownlee (1918) analysed over 100 modern plague epidemics in large towns and presented values of β_1 and β_2.[15] Several of these are given in Table 13 so that the range of values may be seen. He also took four from London in the years 1563, 1603, 1625 and 1665 (these were the earliest epidemics of which sufficient records exist regarding their progress from start to finish). All four curves are very nearly symmetrical. Brownlee had shown that the curve which describes the type of epidemic in many diseases most accurately is the symmetrical form. Commenting upon the symmetry or asymmetry of plague epidemic curves from outbreaks between the Alexandrian epidemic of 1834 and that of Bombay in 1913, Brownlee shows that plague epidemics are as often asymmetrical on the one side as on the other. Thus, the Bombay epidemic of 1905–6, considered in outline, had a decline which was more

TABLE 13

Values of β_1 and β_2 for epidemics of plague in man in large towns (data from Brownlee, 1918)

Town	Date	β_1	β_2
London	1563	0.119	3.222
London	1603	0.032	3.268
London	1625	0.022	3.727
London	1665	0.013	3.488
Alexandria	1834	0.385	5.197
Hong-Kong	1900	0.153	3.855
Sydney	1900	0.001	3.356
Calcutta	1906	0.620	4.097
Bombay	1900	0.006	2.723
Bombay	1909	0.358	4.720
Poonah	1906	0.077	4.373
Belgaum	1897	0.453	3.859

rapid than the rise but when the 16 epidemics in that city between 1898 and 1913 were considered it was seen that whilst those from 1897 to 1906 were similar to the period 1905–06, those from 1906 to 1913 had a decline which was less rapid than the rise. In this type of curve such a configuration might come about if the extension of the epidemic from densely crowded districts to less crowded ones occurred during the decline of the epidemic.

Brownlee considered that owing to the action of chance, asymmetry must occur more or less frequently and that in the outbreaks he studied in large cities, epidemics of plague in man ran a course that was described fairly accurately by the 'epidemic curve' referred to above. A further point of note is that in the crowded city of Bombay with a population of about one million people it took at least four months from the point where the plague-infected *Rattus* increased over the level of the enzootic period to the peak of human deaths. This increase above the off-season enzootic low began in late December in the case of *Rattus rattus* and a little earlier for *Rattus norvegicus*, with the peak of human deaths on 24 April. This was from a situation where plague, to use a modern phrase, arose from a 'flying start' of enzootic plague in the city, rather than from the 'standing start' such as occurred at Messina in Sicily in October 1347. Yet there, according to Ziegler (1970), 'within a few days the plague had taken a firm grasp on the city'.

If the disease was bubonic plague then the few human cases which might have occurred when rats or fleas came ashore would have been followed by a lull which would probably have been longer than Shrewsbury suggests. For any new disease to have taken a hold so quickly it would have needed a more rapid vector mechanism than is available to bubonic plague. Nor is it likely that it was pneumonic plague: as Shrewsbury (1971) says, this needs primary bubonic plague first and that would have taken time to develop before the pneumonic form began to spread.

Any attempt at analysis of epidemic outbreaks during 1348–9 must take into account Brownlee's reluctance to go back earlier than 1563 in his studies on curve qualities. The records of plague deaths in modern epidemics are accurate because diagnosis was improved to such an extent that after 1890 it was unlikely that other illnesses would be confused with plague. However, it is extremely unlikely that diagnosis of the cause of death in the London outbreaks of 1563, 1603, 1625 and 1665 was of such efficiency that counts of plague deaths were totally accurate. It seems more likely that in the confusion and haste to get rid of corpses many deaths from other causes would have been ascribed to plague. The possibilities of comparing epidemic curves in the fourteenth century in the same mathematical terms as those used in the twentieth century are, therefore, remote but a knowledge of such curves may nevertheless offer some guidance.

We have, then, to look at things in a different way when we study the outbreaks of 1348–9. Despite the obvious doubts about diagnosis it is known that a certain number of people died in epidemic circumstances over and above the usual death rate and that this higher mortality extended over a certain period of time. It also occurred at a specific time of year and affected a certain proportion of the total population and it is from this sort of information that we have to make our comparisons.

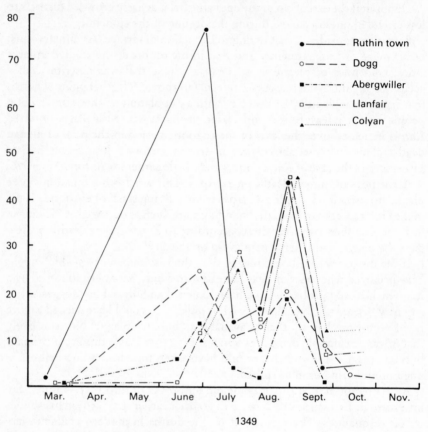

Fig. 14 Deaths in the Lordship of Ruthin, 1349

In Figure 14 I have plotted the deaths from alleged plague in the Lordship of Ruthin during 1349–50 (Rees, 1923) and certain aspects deserve some attention. We have seen already (Chapter 4) that as early as March 1349, an epidemic disease was active in the Lordship of Abergavenny but this would be too early for bubonic plague on climatic evidence, apart from any other reasons. The mortality curves have some features in common. Firstly, each district has two maxima, those of Ruthin Town, Abergwiller and Dogg being in late June and late August, whilst in Llanfair and Colyan the first peak occurred later, around 20 July, but the second peaks coincided with those of the other three areas. It seems improbable that the mortality figures given so precisely by Rees actually occurred on the dates he gives, it is more likely that

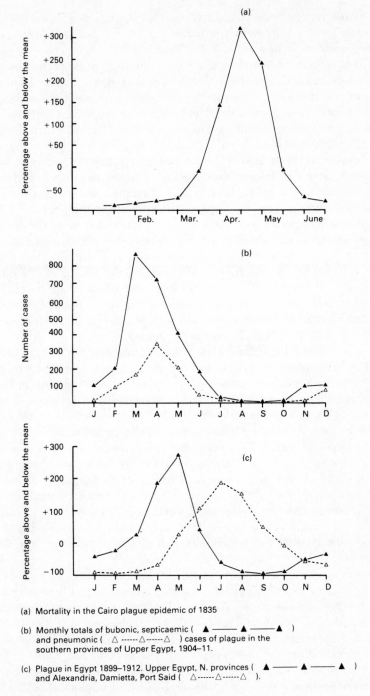

(a) Mortality in the Cairo plague epidemic of 1835

(b) Monthly totals of bubonic, septicaemic (▲ ——— ▲ ——— ▲)
and pneumonic (△ ------△------△) cases of plague in the
southern provinces of Upper Egypt, 1904–11.

(c) Plague in Egypt 1899–1912. Upper Egypt, N. provinces (▲ ——— ▲ ——— ▲)
and Alexandria, Damietta, Port Said (△------△------△).

Fig. 15 Plague in Egypt

the figures represent the cumulative total for the period since the last record. As such, they disguise weekly mortality figures and these would have helped us to see the more subtle changes in death rate.

The question of whether a double mortality peak occurs in plague epidemics seems to have received little attention. As can be seen from Figure 13 the curves for *Rattus rattus* and for man show a double peak but the trough in the human cases is quite small and merely interrupts an otherwise steady upward progression. In the case of the curves for Ruthin Town, Dogg and Abergwiller, there is a fall in the death rate to a low level before the second peak occurs and in the first two areas the initial peak is the greater of the two. The very close similarity of the curves for Llanfair and Colyan and the fact that their first peak occurs later than the first peak of the other three areas inclines one to the view that factors unlike those operating in Ruthin Town, Dogg and Abergwiller were responsible for the first wave of the disease. In other words, in such a small area it is inconceivable that climatic factors could have produced two early peaks three weeks apart since no other aspect of plague biology is so effective in determining the timing of the onset of epidemics. If the late August peaks were the result of the same disease organism and if that same disease had had an earlier peak of deaths, it is unlikely that both of the earlier peaks were also due to plague, one or other was very likely the result of some other disease.

In any case, it is highly improbable that the first peak would have occurred so early in the year. From the Indian experience, the rat epizootic would have had to be at a peak about ten to 14 days earlier, i.e. by the middle of June. In Bombay, with high temperature and humidity, the rat epizootic had been increasing for two and a half months; in Wales this would therefore have begun by early April and flea breeding would have run parallel with it. There are no biological grounds for supporting this contention. There was clearly some disease present but little to support the belief that it was bubonic plague.

The single curve is usually seen in plague epidemics, a good example being the Cairo outbreak of 1835 (Fig. 15a). This shows data for a single epidemic but the other curves for the seasonal prevalence of various types of plague in Egypt (Fig. 15b,c) also show a smooth outline and evidence of a double peak would appear even in this presentation if the disease appeared at various times of the year.

Figure 16 shows the Institutions to vacant benefices in various dioceses during 1348–9 (after Shrewsbury, 1971). Earlier (p. 93), I have pointed out that the peak effects of the disease in England occurred when the disease reached an area, being sometimes in March (February) as in the diocese of Salisbury, April (March) in Exeter or July (June) in Hereford. Commenting on the suggestion by Lunn (1937) that the peak of the epidemic in the Salisbury diocese occurred in February, Shrewsbury says: 'He may be right; but his suggestion runs counter to the usual epidemiological behaviour of bubonic plague in a temperate climate.'

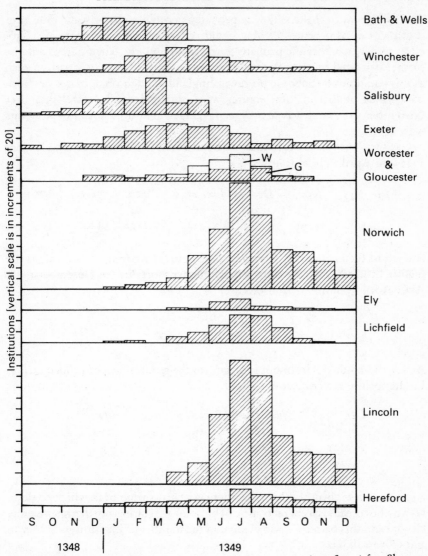

Fig. 16 Seasonal mortality shown by Institutions to vacant benefices (after Shrewsbury, 1971)

Further interesting information is given by Creighton (1894) who showed that during eight months of 1349 the wills are ten or 15 times more numerous than in any other year except perhaps 1361 (the year of the *pestis secunda*). The probate figures he quotes are as follows:

Nov. 1348	Dec.	Jan. 1349	Feb.	Mar.	Apr.	May
3	0	18	42	41	0	121

June	Jly.	Aug.	Sept.	Oct.	Nov.
31	51	0	0	18	27

179

The first point to make is that as probate is not granted for some time after death a peak of probates in May could reflect an April mortality. It is not clear, either, whether the probate courts met regularly. The figures could be further distorted by irregular meetings. In any case, a mortality pattern such as this could not be bubonic plague in England. Creighton does not say from which part of Britain these figures were obtained and he states that after November 1349 there was an ordinary average but he does not show what this was.

Gasquet (1908) lists the number of Institutions in Dorset between October 1348 and April 1349 as follows:

Oct. 1348	Nov.	Dec.	Jan. 1349	Feb.	Mar.	Apr.
5	15	17	16	14	10	4
(4)	(17)	(28)	(21)	(12)	(12)	(6)

and whilst Fletcher (1922) corrected these figures (in parentheses), it alters the picture little other than making a much higher mortality for December 1348. After April 1349 the Institutions are:

May	June	Jly.	Aug.
9	3	11	5

Again, this could not be bubonic plague for the reasons I have outlined earlier. In Hampshire the Institutions were:

Dec. 1348	Jan. 1349	Feb.	Mar.	Apr.
7	12	19	33	46
May	June	Jly.	Aug.	Sept.
29	24	18	11	12

Again, and less abruptly this time, there is a clear spring peak which could in no way be considered characteristic of bubonic plague in a northern temperate climate and this pattern is also evident in the number of Institutions in Devon and Cornwall, viz:

Nov. 1348	Dec.	Jan. 1349	Feb.	Mar.	Apr.
10	6	30	34	60	53
May	June	Jly.	Aug.	Sept.	
47	45	37	16	23	

and, finally, Somerset:

Nov. 1348	Dec.	Jan. 1349	Feb.	Mar.	Apr.	May.	June
9	32	47	43	36	40	21	7

The Institutions and wills show clearly the variation in the timing of the peak mortality and because this is so variable it provides a strong argument against bubonic plague. The fact that there were peaks at different times may be evidence for the presence of more than one epidemic disease. It could also explain why the shapes of the curves do have some differences one from another but it would probably be unwise to attempt to infer too much from that fact alone. I have earlier discussed the possible lag period between the death of an incumbent and the Institution on a short-term basis. There is a further possibility that if disease and death occurred during the summer an appointment might not have taken place before the next winter since patrons often let livings lapse for some time.

Russell (1948) has presented data on the mortality of the population as a whole over the period 1340 to 1500 and compared the pre- and post-plague patterns (Fig. 17). Before the Black Death (1340–7) the heaviest mortality was in January–February and again in October–November. However, his conclusions on this point must be viewed with caution because the total number of deaths for the 12-month period is 159 and that is for a span of *eight* years. When this sample is plotted in graph form (Fig. 17a) it is not quite as simple a picture as Russell suggests for there is a peak in April (15), not quite so high as February (18) but almost the same as January (16). With the exception of March (9) it might be better to speak of a winter and early spring high mortality which ends in May. There is then a relatively low period in June (7) and July (6) and although it is true that October (19) and November (18) have the highest figures in the second half of the year it would be more accurate to suggest that they are the highest points of an increasing mortality which began in August (15) and carried through September (13). There is, from these figures, clear evidence of a higher mortality from August to November inclusive. But this was before the plague so that if bubonic plague came later and produced a heavy mortality in late summer, i.e. August and September after suitable conditions for flea breeding, it would be difficult to separate this from the pre-plague picture.

Looking further at Russell's figures, we turn next to the seven epidemic years in the period 1348–75. These were 1348–50 (but plague did not appear until late 1348), 1360–1, 1369 and 1374. In these years (Fig. 17b) the death rate is only four in January and then begins to increase almost sixfold by February and then steadily to reach an August peak of 75 and then fall to 18 by December. This would be most unlikely to represent a bubonic plague pattern and it would be important to know whether each of the seven years showed the same pattern. According to Russell these seven years accounted for about 20 per cent more deaths than the other 21 years. He says further that the pattern of the mortality shows that plague was severe in August and October with slightly fewer dying in September and claims that so many near the border line of life and death were killed that few of this class were left to die before the next spring. When the figures are plotted (Fig. 17b) the impression

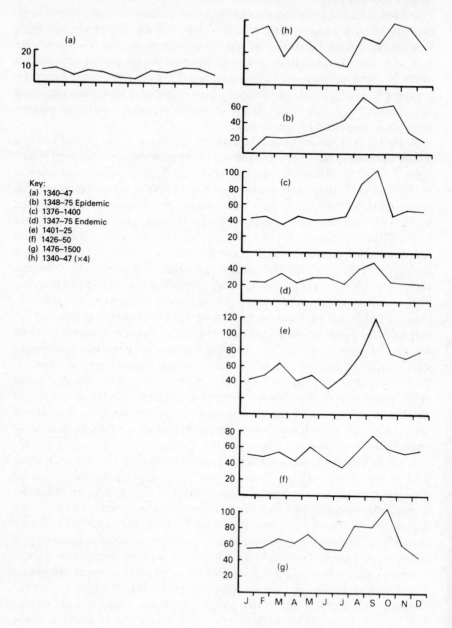

Fig. 17 Monthly mortality for the pre-plague period 1340–7 (a) and for six post-plague periods (b, c, d, e, f, g) (data from Russell, 1948)

given by Russell of a sudden plague epidemic and high mortality in the months stated is seen to be erroneous and August, September and October are seen to be the high months of an increasing mortality which had been gathering pace since as early as February and which by December had not subsided to the January level. It looks as though a disease was active for most of the years but it is unlikely to have been bubonic plague.

Russell then says that the pattern of non-epidemic years was so markedly different from pre-plague and later post-plague periods that the Black Death appears to have been endemic as well as epidemic. He says of the endemic years that there was a July–August high mortality with a level mortality for the rest of the year and cites the period 1376–1400 (Fig. 17c) as an example of this with a slight epidemic amid a general endemic condition of plague. He also selects the non-epidemic, i.e. endemic, years in the period 1347–75 (Fig. 17d). Contrary to what Russell says in the text the figures show the peak mortality months as August and September. At first sight the late summer peaks in curves (c) and (d) appear to support Russell's hypothesis of a short summer epidemic of plague in a general endemic condition. However, if we calculate the percentage of the annual mortality which the summer peak comprises, we find that the late summer/early autumn (August–November) mortality peak in the years 1340–7 accounted for 40 per cent of the years' deaths whilst in the endemic years of 1347–75 the August/September deaths made up 25 per cent, and in the period 1376–1400 almost 30 per cent. It is true that a four monthly period is used in 1340–7 but it is likely that those four months are part of the same heavy death rate and there are no grounds for separating August/September from the yet higher mortality of October/November. Looking at the death rates proportionately, the increase in deaths between July and October, the highest point of the peak in 1340–7, is ×3.2, whereas between July and the highest point (September) in 1347–75 and 1376–1400 is ×2.2 and ×2.3 respectively.

Curve (e) for 1401–25 exhibits a March minor peak (as also did curve (d), 1347–75 endemic years) and a pronounced September peak in which the peak was approximately four times that of the June low mortality. Despite a fall to October, the mortality remained at a high level for the rest of the year and was increasing in December. Curve (f) for 1426–50 also shows a low summer mortality, this time in July, with a September high point and ends in December at the same level as January. Curve (g) for 1476–1500 shows a spring peak from March to May and a higher peak from August to October with a high point in October.

I suggest, therefore, that the mortality patterns in the post-1348 period, whether of epidemic or endemic years, are not sufficiently different from the pre-1348 years as to allow us to believe that bubonic plague was present. Furthermore, the dramatic heights of post-1347 peaks are merely due to the fact that larger numbers are involved: if the curve (a) is scaled up by multiplying by four then it is closely similar to the others (see curve (h)).

That there was heavy mortality from 1348 onwards there seems little doubt. This information from Russell merely serves to show that there was little difference in the pre- and post-1348 mortality patterns except that from 1348 onwards more people died at the same times as before. This could also be interpreted to mean simply that more people were starving to death.

In Figure 5 I have plotted the replacements to benefices in the dioceses of Lincoln and York in the period April 1349 to March 1350 (from Thompson, 1911, 1914). From this it appears that the peak of the epidemic in the six southern archdeaconries of the diocese of Lincoln occurred in July (141) with August (106) as the second highest month. These, however, were part of a high mortality which had probably showed early signs of increase by May and which was still active in November. Thompson unfortunately does not provide a set of control figures for the pre-epidemic period on a monthly basis although he does give the totals. These cover three periods: (a) the 18 months from 23 September 1347 to 24 March 1349; (b) the 12 months from 25 March 1349 to 24 March 1350; and (c) a nine month period from 25 March 1350 to 31 December 1350 and are shown in Table 14.

TABLE 14

Institutions to benefices in the diocese of Lincoln in the pre-epidemic period 23 September 1347–24 March 1349, during the epidemic 25 March 1349–24 March 1350 and following the epidemic 25 March 1350–31 December 1350

Archdeaconry	23 September, 1347 to 24 March, 1349 (18 months)	25 March, 1349 to 24 March, 1350 (12 months)	25 March, 1350 to 31 December, 1350 (9 months)
Lincoln	62	280	7
Stow	6	66	4
Bedford	4	52	7
Buckingham	13	77	1
Huntingdon	13	66	3
Leicester	19	84	9
Northampton	11	130	7
Oxford	6	70	3
TOTAL	134	825	41

In the two northern archdeaconries of Lincoln and Stow the months of July and August had very similar death rates or, more correctly, Institutions to vacant benefices, but the peak period was prolonged in relation to the southern archdeaconries. In the diocese of York the peak period of Institutions was in September, with October also high. As Figure 5 shows, the mortality pattern in York was somewhat different from the other two in having a much less rapid increase to the peak. Between the two Lincoln curves that of the south has both a steeper rise, which begins earlier, and a more rapid decline than the northern one. As Lunn (1937; in Shrewsbury) has pointed out in relation to Salisbury diocese so Thompson (1911) also points out that it is obvious that the daily Institutions which took place in June, July and August did not follow very quickly upon the voidance of the benefices; and that the statistics to be obtained from those months actually refer to a period a few weeks, at any rate, before their date. This factor has not been adequately emphasised in the analyses of plague mortality based on Institutions. The difficulty arises of knowing how far behind actual deaths the Institutions lagged. Lunn suggested one month. If this is done in Figure 5 (dotted line) it would be even less likely that rat breeding, flea breeding and the climate could all have been sufficiently active to promote plague. Even without any adjustment the peak in July would be too early for an epidemic (and preceding epizootic) of plague arising from an existing enzootic situation, let alone an epidemic which would have had to spread *de novo*. By correcting for the lag between death and Institution, the earlier peak would be an impossibility for bubonic plague.

The disease would be expected to have spread northwards from the counties of East Anglia, which it had reached in May 1349, spreading through the rat population and causing local epizootics. Yet throughout this large area the high mortality occurred only one month later over the whole diocese. Plague is said to have reached York on 21 May but according to Thompson (1914) the deaths of clergy over the whole of this vast northern diocese were on the increase soon afterwards. As we have seen, bubonic plague can be excluded from the reckoning if these facts are correct, and there is no reason to doubt them. In view of the widespread and almost simultaneous mortality the organism responsible appears more likely to have been an air-borne pathogen spread by respiratory means.

The seasonal mortality pattern during the Black Death must be one of the most telling arguments against it being bubonic plague. Levett (1938), in an account of the epidemic on the St Albans Manors, showed that the majority of deaths were reported at the spring courts held in April and May 1349. For example, in the manor of Codicote the majority, 59, occurred between 1 November 1348 and 19 May 1349, only six deaths being recorded after May 1349. In Cashio the worst, 55 deaths, was over by 3 May, 18 dying after that date. In the manor of Langley also, the court on 1 May 1349 recorded 73 deaths with only nine in the autumn court of 1348. In Norton there were four deaths between the autumn court of 1348 and 25 April, but 20 between that date and 29 June.

Levett comments that the violence of the epidemic was exhausted before the summer began and that corroborative evidence may be discovered elsewhere to show that from February to the middle or end of May would cover the period of greatest danger, this being particularly true of the eastern and east-midland counties.

Shrewsbury also comments upon this unexpected pattern. For example, Parliament in London was prorogued on 1 January 1349 as a result of a sudden pestilence at Westminster. It was prorogued again on 10 March and Shrewsbury says that it seems evident that plague was active in London during the winter months, an occurrence he considered unusual because of the fact that in temperate latitudes the rat fleas would usually hibernate with the onset of cold, frosty weather, and plague would thus be extinguished or become quiescent. He considers there is evidence to suggest that 'The Great Pestilence' may have been an exception to this rule, because if only a half of the excessive number of vacant benefices in the diocese of Salisbury during the autumn of 1348 and the winter of 1349 was caused by the deaths of their incumbents from bubonic plague, the disease must have been continuously active in Dorsetshire, Wiltshire and Berkshire throughout those seasons. Despite the claims that the autumn of 1348 and the winter of 1349 were exceptionally mild, it seems to be a case of adjusting the disease to fit events atypical of its pattern, especially as, elsewhere, Shrewsbury says that plague has not changed its epidemiological character during the period of recorded history.

The winters may have been mild but they appear to have been very wet also. Titow (1959-60) shows that the whole of 1348 and 1349 was wet (there is no information on the summer of 1348) with flooding reported in winter, 1348 and winter and autumn, 1349. These conditions would not seem to be ideal for the spread of bubonic plague.

As we know from field studies, in order to initiate epidemics of bubonic plague there must be an extensive rat population in fairly close proximity to

TABLE 15

Relationship between plague infection and population size in Indian communities (after Greenwood, 1910)

Mean population	% never infected	% infected once	% infected twice	% infected 3 times	% infected 4 or more times
92	80	20	0	0	0
257	51	32	17	0	0
352	50	33	14	0	0
603	31	32	32	5	0
784	21	39	35	5	0
1059	15	34	46	2	3
1465	7	25	61	7	0
2373	5	15	64	15	0

man, with enzootic plague alternating with the epizootic state in the rats and thereby producing human cases. The Black rat is for good reason known as the House rat, particularly in temperate latitudes, and it is unrealistic to think of plague as an essentially rural disease. Even in India this has been seen to be true. Greenwood (1910) analysed epidemics of bubonic plague in three districts of the Punjab and concluded that there was a direct relationship between the number of epidemics in which villages had been attacked and the average population of such villages. The average population of villages which had never been attacked was very small: of villages with a mean population of 92, 80 per cent were never infected and 20 per cent were infected only once, and of villages with a mean population of 352, 50 per cent were never infected and 33 per cent only infected once (Table 15). Plague could maintain itself in towns but not to any extent in villages unless they were large.

It has been said that 90 per cent of the population of fourteenth-century England lived in villages. Russell (1948), in an analysis of the distribution of the population of England, defined the various sized communities as follows:

Small hamlet	1–25
Hamlet	26–50
Small village	51–100
Village	101–200
Small market town	201–400
Large market town	401–800

His analysis covered 21 counties or parts of counties in 1377 and showed a total of 4264 communities. Looking at Table 16 it is seen that 60 per cent of the total number of settlements contained between 51 and 200 people each. However, a small number of large settlements might be more important than many small communities in maintaining plague or its vectors. As can be seen from Table 16 the number of people in 401–800 sized units is 96,000, almost the same as in 51–100 sized units but in the latter case they are distributed in 1261 settlements whilst in the former only 160. Russell also shows that the distribution of settlement sizes varies from one region to another and whilst Northumberland, out of 157 communities, had only 13 (8.3 per cent) with more than 100 persons, Kent had 80 (38 per cent) out of 210. Thus, if what Greenwood (1910) said about Indian communities held good for Britain then one would expect plague not only to fail to become established in the vast majority of communities but also fail to even attack them. Yet despite this evidence and that presented earlier concerning the biology of the rat and flea, it is said that plague in its first visitation was characterised by a universality of incidence and it was this that chiefly distinguished the Black Death from the later outbreaks which differed by being more often in towns than villages or solitary houses and were also rarely in many places in the same year (Creighton, 1894).

It is generally believed that bubonic plague was very severe on a national scale in the early stages of the current pandemic in India and I have argued

TABLE 16

Distribution of the population of some English counties in 1377 (after Russell, 1948)

Size of settlement	1–25 people	26–50	51–100	101–200	201–400	401–800
Number of settlements (4264)	222	606	1261	1304	711	160
% of total number of settlements	5.2	14.2	29.6	30.6	16.7	3.8
Number of people (taking mid-point of size)	2662	22,422	94,575	195,600	213,300	96,000
% of total number of people	0.43	3.59	15.1	31.3	34.2	15.4

against this elsewhere. Even when viewed at the village level the Indian experience shows that when one looks at actual plague deaths the figure is not high when expressed as a proportion of the total population although it may be quite high as a proportion of the annual number of deaths. For example, in the village of Parel, near Bombay, a community of 3525 people (called a village but about the same size as Oxford in 1377) during the 12 months from November 1905 to October 1906 inclusive, a total of 90 people died. Twenty-one of these (23 per cent) were plague victims, 12 (13 per cent) died of cholera and the remaining 57 (63 per cent) from a variety of other causes. It is interesting that the peak month for cholera was also one of the two peak plague months, the requirements of the two diseases being similar in regard to temperature in India as they would be in England. When we look at the plague *case mortality* in this village the picture is more stark with 75 per cent of those contracting plague actually dying of the disease. It seems clear that in the course of plague literature there has arisen some confusion between case mortality, plague deaths as a proportion of all deaths and plague deaths as a proportion of the total population of the community. That there is a great deal of difference is obvious but case mortalities and especially plague deaths related to total deaths have all too easily been translated to total population mortality.

Data from some other villages in the neighbourhood of Bombay give good evidence on plague death rates in small settlements (small communities suffered higher plague mortality than larger ones) although it should be noted that these villages were large in comparison with those of fourteenth-century England. A typical case is the village of Dhand (population 2000). Details for three epidemics are given (a) in the period November 1902 to March 1903, (b)

April 1905 and (c) between February and May 1906 (Plague Research Commission, 1907b). The following was recorded:

Period	Number of plague cases	Number dying of plague	Plague case mortality	Plague deaths as percentage of total population
(a)	153	81	52.9	4.05
(b)	47	21	44.7	1.05
(c)	32	19	59.4	0.95

The plague deaths as a percentage of the total population, translated to fourteenth-century English villages, would scarcely have been noticed amidst the plethora of other fatal ailments.

Because of the impossibility of determining the absolute number of plague deaths in 1348–9 the mortality has been calculated as being equivalent to the percentage of Institutions to vacant benefices with further evidence from manorial records and the Inquisitions *Post Mortem*. It may be unwise to assume that the death rate of the clergy was equivalent to that in the population as a whole because, as Ziegler points out, despite the fact that beneficed clergy had higher living standards and less cramped living conditions, they might actually have had a higher death rate than the laity because their calling would bring them into contact with infected people. Ziegler maintains that where pulmonary plague was present it was a death sentence. However, modern evidence does not wholeheartedly support this contention and in the case of bubonic plague there may be very little risk in visiting the patient. Because the average age of the clergy was probably higher than that of the population as a whole, in any year a higher proportion of priests was likely to die and whilst one may agree with Ziegler on this point it is less easy to agree with his assumption that whilst the smaller size of a priest's household may have reduced the chances of infection (he does not say how), 'it seems also to have been the case that, once such a household was infected, the chances of any survivals were proportionately less'. As I have said earlier there is no basis for the numbers of rats and fleas per English household which Ziegler presents with the conclusion that 'the greater the number of infected fleas in proportion to potential human victims, the smaller the chances of escape'. Although this might be reasonably expected there is little evidence to support it and even when we look at major plague zones such as Mandui, a plague area of Bombay with an average of 3.1 *plague* rats per building, the average number of human plague deaths in each building was 0.6 (Plague Research Commission, 1907b; Hirst, 1953). I have elsewhere (Chapter 9) shown that in India there were more fleas per rat than the three assumed by Ziegler to be the quota on English rats.

The first half of the fourteenth century was a period of instability. Ennen

(1979) says that the population curve altered in the fourteenth century and as evidence of this negative trend points to the frequency of abandoned settlements in the countryside, the pause in the eastward colonisation by peasants in Europe, the abandonment of new town foundations and arrested growth in many established towns leading to a marked decline in urban populations. She points out that in many cases the population decline had begun before the Black Death of 1348 and that the epidemic was only a part of the phenomenon. Ennen considers that because the medieval mortality rate was so high, a small reduction in the birth rate was sufficient to cause a population reduction and suggests that the famines of 1315–17 may have weakened the people so much that it was a contributory factor to the high death rate in 1348–9. When disease closely follows famine then it is likely that the weakened population would succumb but it is difficult to see how the same effect would come about thirty years later.

Bath (1963) subscribed to the view that overpopulation between 1150 and 1300 resulted in a great toll of life by the epidemics of the fourteenth and fifteenth centuries, the high mortality from the Black Death and the other fourteenth-century epidemics being explained by the result of prolonged undernourishment. Elaborating on this theme he claimed that the people of the Dutch coastal areas, who lived mainly from stock-farming and fishery and consequently ate more animal proteins and fats than the arable-farming folk, did not succumb to the fourteenth-century epidemics to anything like the same degree.

Information is now beginning to emerge about the diet of medieval Englishmen and Dr T. P. O'Connor has kindly given me some of the results of excavations. It is his impression from studying medieval food debris that the meat component of the diet was varied and that wild fowl and fish were well exploited. From medieval York there are contemporaneous assemblages from what are probably rich and poor parts of the city. The more prosperous people of Bishophill supplemented their diet with swan and woodcock whilst the poorer people ate pigeon and even guillemot. O'Connor is of the opinion that whilst a cereal failure would have seriously affected the bottom ten per cent of the population, the rest would be capable of adjusting to the situation and even those unable to afford beef and mutton apparently had access to pigeons and eels.

Postan and Titow (1958–9) concluded from their study of heriots (death duties levied on holdings of customary tenants) and prices on five Winchester manors from 1245–1347 that a society where every harvest failure resulted in a large increase in deaths was balanced on the margin of subsistence. Such a balance, which was so often upset, implied one or both of two inter-related possibilities. The first was that cultivation had reached the point where the land could keep those who tilled it only in years of favourable harvests which might be expected in two years out of three. The second possibility was that the holdings were so small that they could only support their cultivators in years of good harvests. The conclusion from this was that there was rural over-population, the numbers of peasants on the land being greater than its produce could support. Many factors probably contributed to the population reduction over a period of several years and the epidemic of 1348–9 doubtless assisted the decline.

It is difficult to determine which age classes were differentially susceptible to the medieval epidemic and whether there was any bias towards one sex or another. Russell (1948) says of the second plague of 1361 that it was called the 'mortalite des enfaunz' by one chronicler and that the third plague of 1369 was said by another to have been especially severe on children. He also was of the opinion that plague was most serious to children for he says that while the plague was the cause of marked population changes the loss was more that of high infant and child mortality than of an equal incidence among all classes of the population. However, the statistics on the age incidence of bubonic plague in India scarcely bear this out and the findings of high child mortality in these epidemics might prove a pointer to the presence of one or more other diseases active at that time.

Russell finds no evidence of any difference in mortality rate between men and women although from the following remarks he clearly expected to: 'The problem of the mortality of women is obviously important, since they included half of the population. Because the Black Death attacked the glands, it might be expected that men, *since they have more glands*, (my italics) might have been more severely affected with a higher death rate as a result. There seems no evidence that it was much higher'. Just which glands Russell had in mind is not clear. So far as I can find there is no evidence that men have more lymph glands than women and the only extra glands which men have are those associated with the male reproductive system and these have no part in plague infections. This statement is a good example of how some contributors to the plague literature have often not fully understood the disease.

It seems, then, that with the exception of the relatively few urban centres, bubonic plague would have been unlikely to have become established in fourteenth-century northern Europe with its scattered, small communities in which lived most of the population. Within densely crowded towns nearer to the Mediterranean or even in a few more northerly towns when local conditions favoured the maintenance of Black rat colonies and in hot summers there could have been the opportunity for bubonic plague to have arisen. I have already indicated my doubts about rapid spread because of the dissected nature of towns but where large numbers of inhabitants lived crowded in the same building as was common in cities of southern Europe then the increase in density per unit area might favour the spread of epidemic diseases. Ennen (1979) gives some interesting figures on the population density in some medieval towns, unfortunately no British ones. The density was much greater in the south of Europe with Genoa having 545 persons per hectare and Toulon 500 compared with Brussels with 56 and Bruges at 81 per hectare.

Seeing that the bulk of the population of England during the fourteenth century lived in villages, it would have been instructive to have been able to follow an epidemic of the Great Pestilence in a village community. This, unfortunately, is not possible because there was no detailed record of deaths in a parish and it was not until parish registers were used that an accurate record of population changes was made. Thus I have turned to a supposed outbreak of plague in a village during the seventeenth century as an alternative.

Plague is said to have remained in the British Isles until the late seventeenth century and many outbreaks of disease have been documented under this heading. In some of the later ones there are accurate mortality data from which epidemic curves can be plotted. An example of one such is from the village of Eyam in the Peak District of Derbyshire in 1665 and 1666. The village at the onset of the epidemic contained about 350 inhabitants, forming a rural community at an altitude of around 800 feet above sea level. The winters are frequently marked by heavy snowfalls as the village lies at the southern end of the Pennines and has a fairly high annual precipitation. There is some mixed farming but the land is not good and the summers are too wet to suit cereal crops. Most land is pasture and milk the main agricultural product along with sheep farming on the nearby heather moors. Many village people work in the nearby limestone quarries. In this bleak environment it is impossible to believe that *Rattus rattus* could have survived if introduced, let alone have formed a widespread population.

The story of plague in the village in the years 1665–6 has received much attention from local and national historians and proves a strong tourist attraction. In his book on Eyam, Wood (1865) discusses the history of plague and in great detail documents the deaths of the villagers. He says of the Black Death that it 'was characterized by copious hemorrhage'. This is interesting, and the first modern mention of such a symptom so far as I can find. It would not be thought to be characteristic of bubonic plague today. He goes on:

> it was, however, divested of this awfully fatal symptom, that the plague was brought by some ships from Cyprus or Candia, in the Levant, to Amsterdam and Rotterdam, where it made terrible carnage in the year 1663. Two Frenchmen are said to have brought it in some woollen goods from Holland to London, in December, 1664. These two Frenchmen, who resided in Longacre, London, on opening their goods, were seized with the plague, and, in a day or two, died in great agonies. Thus began, in London, this terrible scourge, which from December, 1664, to the beginning of 1666, carried off 100,000 souls.

From what Wood says, it appears that the haemorrhage was not present in this epidemic. It may, however, be of interest that the disease was thought to have arisen from contact with woollen goods, since it is said that the plague reached Eyam in late 1665 by the same means. According to Dr Richard Mead, writing in 1744:

the plague was likewise at Eham, in the Peak of Derbyshire; being brought thither, by means of a box sent from London to a taylor in that village, containing some materials relating to his trade. A servant who opened the foresaid box, complaining that the goods were damp, was ordered to dry them by the fire; but in so doing it was seized with the plague and died.

This first burial took place on 7 September 1665, the next on 22 September with another four before the end of the month. October saw 23 dead, November seven and December nine. Wood comments that whilst the great plague in London appeared in the latter end of 1664 and was checked by the winter, at Eyam, 'where the effects of winter would be considerably greater than in cities, the plague continued its ravages without ceasing'.

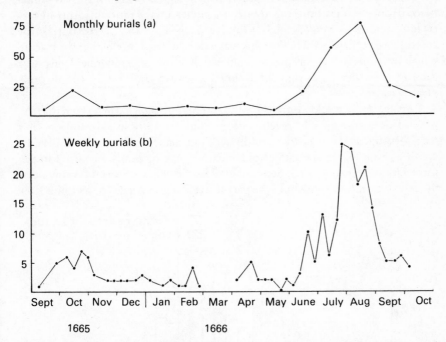

Fig. 18 Mortality of the inhabitants of the village of Eyam in the Peak District of Derbyshire: September 1665–October 1666.

Figure 18 shows the burials for the period September 1665 to October 1666. As can be seen, there was a steady monthly death rate from September 1665 until May 1666 except for the higher October 1665 figure. If we look at curve (a) where only the monthly total of burials is plotted, it can be seen that the peak death rate occurs in August 1666. The difficulty with monthly figures is in deciding where in the month to place them; they may be useful in some treatments but in the case of epidemics a shorter time unit is essential. As the dates of burials in Eyam are known, they can be plotted on a weekly basis, curve (b), and this somewhat alters the picture.

Going back to the start of the epidemic the monthly figures for burials show an almost fourfold increase between September and October but the weekly burials show that the deaths occurred at a fairly high level of around five to seven per week from the last week in September to the beginning of November. By mid-November the burials were down to two a week and remained at that level until the end of December. Although the burials per month were low from November to the end of May, in comparison with what was to come in the summer of 1666, they would nevertheless appear high in relation to Wood's estimate of the total population of about 350. The average of 'non-plague' months was very nearly seven per month. Assuming a similar death rate for the whole year this would be 84 per annum; in other words 25 per cent of the population dying each year. Even allowing for the ills which beset people at that time together with higher infant mortality this nevertheless appears to be very high. Only an analysis of pre-plague burials for several years will show whether this was a normal level or whether the disease which was alleged to be plague and which came in September 1665 was causing extra deaths during the following winter and spring, i.e. at 'non-plague' times.

Turning to the weekly burials for the summer of 1666 it can be seen that the peak of the epidemic was reached during the last week in July and the first week of August. This contrasts oddly with the data for the London mortality in 1665 (Fig. 19). In the latter epidemic the peak of deaths occurred in the three weeks beginning on 5 September. This, in the warmer environment of the city of London where bubonic plague may have existed, was a month later

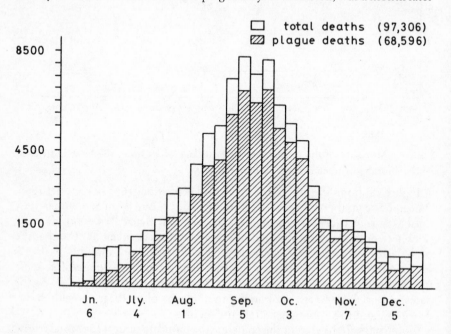

Fig. 19 Total deaths and plague deaths in London, 1665

than in the cooler climate of a Pennine village. In London, plague deaths rose from a very low level at the end of May and reached an epidemic peak three months later. In Eyam, with a much more scattered population, the peak was reached seven weeks after the low period of the first week in June.

According to Shrewsbury, plague deaths were still occurring in London as late as 19 December 1665 and in Figure 19 is shown the plague deaths in each month from December 1665 to November 1666. This indicates that plague increased in January 1666 and was active throughout the winter months. It would be interesting to know how winter cases of plague were identified, since there would be little likelihood of bubonic plague being present and pneumonic plague would be indistinguishable in those days from any other respiratory ailment. There would appear to have been plenty of cases of plague after 22 November, despite the entry in Pepys' diary for that date in which he observed that the death-roll was decreasing and that there were 'great hopes of a further decrease, because of this day's being a very exceeding hard frost, and continues freezing' (Mynors Bright, 1953).

According to Wood, 76 per cent of the population of Eyam died[16] in the period under discussion but this estimate has been questioned on various points (Bradley, 1977). In the Bombay epidemic of 1905–6 a total of 9210 people died of plague in the 12 months, out of a total population of nearly one million. Petrie and Todd (1923) point out that the numbers dying of plague in Egypt were small when compared with Indian outbreaks where the deaths alone in each of the first ten epidemics in the city of Bombay ranged from 10,000 to 20,000. But a toll of 20,000 lives out of one million inhabitants represents a death rate of 2.0 per cent and the percentage dying of plague in the 1905–6 epidemic would therefore be 0.9 per cent of the total population of Bombay. I have elsewhere quoted the Egyptian data from the Kôm Ombo epidemic in which 1.8 per cent of the population died of plague and the overall plague deaths in Egypt over 20 years from which 0.007 per cent of the population died of plague per annum.

The total number of deaths from all causes in London in the year 1665 was 97,306, of which 68,596 were said to be due to plague. Shrewsbury accepts 350,000 as the maximum population in London in 1636 and taking this as a starting point, then 27.8 per cent of the population died in 1665 and 19.6 per cent died of plague. Brett-James (1935) considered that the population had risen to 460,000. If that was so then the corresponding death rates would be 21.2 per cent and 14.9 per cent, still a high proportion of the total population.

In Table 17 I have calculated the annual deaths from plague as a percentage of the total population figure. The majority of records used are from the current pandemic between 1896 and 1919, and for Asian countries and Egypt where plague was severe. The highest percentage, excluding Europe, was 0.305 in Ceylon. These figures contrast markedly with the Black Death in England where estimates of mortality vary between 30 and 50 per cent and even with the London epidemic of 1665.

TABLE 17

Percentage of total population dying of plague per annum

Country/Town	Years	Plague deaths	Plague deaths per annum	Total population	% total population dying of plague per annum
India	1896–1917	9,841,396	447,336	329,000,000	0.135
Ceylon	1914–1917	978	244	800,000	0.305
Straits Settlements	1910–1917	280	40	1,000,000	0.004
Dutch East Indies	1911–1917	34,732	5,788	40,000,000	0.014
Siam	1911–1917	1,063	177	9,000,000	0.0019
French Indo-China	1911–1917	14,911	2,485	18,000,000	0.0138
Hongkong	1895–1917	15,731	715	520,000	0.138
Japan	1907–1916	1,380	153	50,000,000	0.00031
Formosa	1896–1917	24,108	1,095	3,400,000	0.032
Egypt	1899–1919	14,783	739	11,200,000+	0.007
London	1665	68,596	–	350,000–460,000	14.9–19.6
England	1348–1350	1.3–2.0 million	–	–	30.0–50.0 in total
Eyam (Derbyshire)	Sept. 1665 –Oct. 1666 incl.	266	–	c. 350	76.0 in 14 months (But see Bradley, 1977)

It is generally held that after the initial, very high mortality in the Black Death, the death rate became less as the population became resistant. It is interesting, therefore, to examine this aspect of the disease pattern and the early years of this century in India provide such a situation. Seal (1969) examined the period 1898–1957 and, taking the era as a series of roughly ten-year periods, showed that plague mortality, expressed as a rate per 100,000 people, declined with each ten-year spell, e.g.

1898–1908 inclusive	–	183.3 per 100,000
1908–1918 inclusive	–	133.8 per 100,000
1919–1928 inclusive	–	51.9 per 100,000

up to the last nine years (1949–57) when it was only 1.8 per 100,000. This method, however, disguises the annual mortality. Seal presents a diagram which shows plague mortality in India per 100,000 of the population in each year from 1897 onwards, and although it is only a histogram without exact figures a fairly accurate estimate can be made of the deaths. It shows that in the first 11 years of plague the following death rates occurred:

Year	Plague deaths/100,000
1897	c. 20
1898	c. 35
1899	c. 50
1900	c. 35
1901	c. 100
1902	c. 180
1903	c. 270
1904	c. 370
1905	c. 340
1906	c. 115
1907	c. 410

Clearly, the effect was not an immediate, heavy mortality such as was claimed in Britain in 1348–9 and it was as long as 11 years before the highest death rate was reached. During the first four years 50 plague deaths per 100,000 of the population was the maximum attained. This would be 500 per million and the same rate translated to 1348 would represent about 2000 out of a population of four million. Even after 11 years of plague in India the peak of 410 per 100,000 would only be 16,400 in four million yet the claims for the effect of the Black Death vary from 1,300,000 (30 per cent) to two million (50 per cent).

After this peak in 1907 in India the plague death rate per annum fell steadily with lesser peaks in 1911 (c. 250 per 100,000), 1918 (200 per 100,000) and 1924 (125 per 100,000). Because the number of plague deaths was high in the first 11 years in India (over 6,000,000) we are tempted to think that a large proportion of the population died but in fact when we consider that this is just over 540,000 per annum out of a total population at that time of 329 million people it is seen to be very low.

Shrewsbury has produced some rather inaccurate estimates of death rates from bubonic plague. He says, 'In most of the urban outbreaks in India resulting from the last pandemic of the disease which erupted in 1898, about one-third of the population was attacked, with a case-mortality rate ranging from 70 to 80 per cent, giving an absolute mortality rate that did not exceed one-quarter of the population.' In other words, about 98 million people were infected, of which 70 to 80 million died; this contrasts markedly with the official statistics where less than ten million died between 1896 and 1917. Shrewsbury is correct in his observations that between 70 and 80 per cent of plague cases died in India but the real facts are that in the first four years and ten months of plague from September 1896 to late June 1901, there were only 659,864 plague cases out of a population which numbered 294,266,702 at the 1901 census (Low, 1902). Out of this huge population, then, there were on average as few as 132,000 cases per annum.

Other statistics from plague in India are also misleading, e.g. Gill (1928) who purports to show a plague death rate per thousand during the period 1898–1918 for all India of 33.65, whereas the true figure is 3.365. Gill has inflated the death rate in his calculations by taking the mean population for one year but the plague deaths for a 20-year period and calculating rates per thousand on this basis. If calculated on a per annum basis the death rates are better understood and I have attempted to do this in Table 17.

Shrewsbury uses his version of the Indian data to estimate the death rate in London in 1348 when 'The Great Pestilence' arrived in the city saying, 'If its population did not exceed 60,000, a generous estimate of its plague death-roll – based on late nineteenth-century statistics of urban epidemics of bubonic plague in India – would place it between 15,000 and 20,000. Creighton's estimate is that its mortality ranged between 20,000 and 30,000'. As I have shown earlier in this chapter plague epidemics in urban areas such as Bombay have never produced death rates as high as these.

There are inevitably some extraordinarily high estimates of mortality during the Great Pestilence and also some curious inconsistencies in the reporting, the substance of which can make an appreciable difference to our understanding of the severity of the epidemic. For example, Robert of Avesbury's account of events in London in 1349 was that the disease, 'reaching London about the Feast of All Souls, killed many each day, and from the Feast of the Purification (2 February) until after Easter it so increased that almost every day there were buried in the new cemetery, then made at Smithfield, more than 200 bodies of the dead, over and above those buried in the other cemeteries of the city'.[17] This would indicate a severe disease, active during the late winter months. Yet Thompson (1889), in a commentary to the text which he edited, says that between the Purification and Easter 200 bodies were buried in the new burial ground in Smithfield. This version would imply a less severe epidemic. The comment that this estimate contrasts modestly with Stow's assertion that no less than 50,000 persons were buried during the course of a year in that place indicates the very variable nature of mortality estimates. Few were truly reliable and in any case were at best counts of all deaths, whatever the cause.

In the light of these statements it is easy to see how the effects of the great medieval pandemic have been exaggerated. In no part of the world has bubonic plague produced a mortality as high as that claimed in England, where conditions in most respects did not favour this disease. Yet in India where the climate favoured high flea populations and where there were abundant rats, severe human overcrowding and undernourishment, the disease had a relatively low death rate and a slow speed of spread.

Clinical symptoms in the Black Death and in some other diseases. The case for anthrax

It is important to realise that the disease of 1348–50 was one episode out of very many severe epidemics which had afflicted the people of the British Isles since the early part of the sixth century and earlier. Bonser (1944) has analysed the series of epidemics which occurred during the Anglo-Saxon period and the first thing that strikes one is the frequency with which they took place when an epidemic period was under way. Secondly, there were long intervals without any noted epidemics.

During the 6th century A.D. there were disease outbreaks in the years c. 526, 537, 544, 547 ('mortalitas magna' in Britain), 548 (in Ireland), 550, 552, 553, 555. Bonser says of this period that the main affliction appears to have been some cutaneous disease designated 'pestis flava', and MacArthur (1944) in an appendix to Bonser was of the opinion that the disease, also known as the Yellow Pestilence, or *buidhe-conaill*, and often identified with bubonic plague, a view which MacArthur himself had formerly held, was in fact a severe form of relapsing fever with jaundice present often enough to dominate the general picture of the disease. There followed a gap of 109 years and then, beginning in A.D. 664, a series of outbreaks occurred during the next 25 years as follows: 663–7, 672, 676–86, 688 (in 684–6 there was also mortality of animals). These, too, Bonser thought were probably 'pestis flava'.

The various plagues (in the general use of the term) during the ninth to eleventh centuries were considered to be the result of famine and the following shows the frequency of famine, plague and murrain (cattle disease) during this period: 793 (famine), 800 (murrain), 831, 2 or 3 (mortalitas), 868 (famine), 869 (famine, plague and murrain), 897 (plague and murrain), 962 (pestilence), 963 (famine in Ireland), 974 (famine and murrain), 986 (murrain in Ireland), 987 (plague and murrain), 1005 (famine), 1010 (probably dysentery in Danish army in Kent), 1011 (the same in Ireland). During the Confessor's reign the pattern was repeated in various permutations in the years 1041, 1044, 1046, 1047, 1049, 1054, 1063, 1086, 1087. It should perhaps be borne in mind that because of the way in which medieval men looked at history, natural disasters might appear retrospectively during a troubled reign.

Famine was common in people lacking food reserves and one or two poor seasons would be sufficient to create famine conditions which in turn would lead to the famine fevers, principally typhus with varying amounts of relapsing fever, the latter, according to MacArthur (1944), being most evident at the beginning and end of the epidemic. Between 1087 and 1143 the catalogue continued with either famines, pestilence or murrain occurring in 19 of the 56 years (Creighton, 1894). During the fourteenth century there had been several poor harvests, those before 1315 leading to the great famine of 1315, 1316 and 1317 (Lucas, 1930). Lucas records how large numbers of sheep and cattle died and speculates that the great murrain which killed cattle may have been anthrax which killed people who ate the infected flesh. Disease was rife, with dysentery, fever and a fetid throat infection, the latter, from what we know today, probably being diphtheria. MacArthur (1959) says that the whole circumstances of famine allowed smouldering patches of typhus to flare up and spread. There had been bad harvests before 1348 so that typhus was probably active at the same time as the Great Pestilence. This sequence of famine and disease was common and Boucher (1938) says that England experienced ten large-scale visitations of famine and disease in the eleventh century, twelve in the twelfth century and eleven in the thirteenth century. However, when considering typhus as a likely alternative to plague its pattern of alternating febrile and fever-free periods and consequent lengthy period of illness rules it out.

The precise identification of the various epidemics prior to the fourteenth century is difficult and even medically trained men and bacteriologists disagree (Howe, 1972). There is some agreement that typhus and relapsing fever were present and probably smallpox, scurvy and dysentery. Many diseases produce skin reactions and it is likely that some of these have been used as evidence that bubonic plague was present but there is no convincing evidence that this disease occurred in pre-fourteenth-century Britain. Shrewsbury is of this opinion and goes further by saying that even when the record of an ancient pestilence shows ulcerating buboes in the inguinal region it does not identify it as bubonic plague because bubonous ulcers may develop in the groins in fatal cases of confluent smallpox.

Reading the many and varied accounts of the Black Death one is struck by the attempts to highlight those features which support a diagnosis of bubonic plague and to ignore those points which might run counter to the identification of this disease. In pointing this out I am aware that I have to be especially careful in my doubts about the occurrence of bubonic plague not to fall into the same trap in reverse. I intend to draw attention to some features which deserve attention and to explore alternative diseases which might have been present contemporaneous with plague or might even have been the main disease, at least in some areas.

A good starting point is the name Black Death. Gasquet (1908) says that it is a modern term and the disease at the time was called 'the pestilence', 'the great mortality', 'the death', or 'the plague of Florence'. He thinks that 'Black Death' was first used in Denmark or Sweden but was doubtful whether the 'atra mors' of Pontanus (1631) was equivalent to the English Black Death. In England the term was used only after the disease epidemic of the seventeenth century had assumed the title of the Great Plague and Gasquet wondered whether the name was first used to express the state of mourning produced or to mark the *special characteristic symptoms* of this epidemic (the italics are mine). He did not consider it important which of these was the true reason but it is surely of some note that the symptoms of this epidemic were considered to be so unusual. He elaborates this point in describing the symptoms: the disease presented as swellings and carbuncles under the arm and in the groin, these being either few and as large as a hen's egg or smaller and all over the body. In this respect the disease was similar to the later plague of 1665. However, Gasquet then outlines the special symptoms apparent in 1348–9, these being: gangrenous inflammation of the throat and lungs, violent pains in the region of the chest, the vomiting and spitting of blood and the pestilential odour coming from the bodies and breath of the sick.

Gasquet says that the characteristic symptoms of the epidemic, noted in many contemporary accounts (he does not say which), appear to be identical with those of the disease known as malignant pustule of the lung, 'and it would appear probable that this outbreak of plague *must be distinguished from every other of which there is any record*'. I can find no other writer who has mentioned this lung condition. This unique quality of the 1348–9 epidemic is worth noting. So also is the comment by the French physician Anglada (1869) who claimed, 'the Black Death stands apart from all those *which preceded or followed it*. It ought to be classed among the great and new popular maladies'.

Another curious piece of information, which seems to have been over-looked, is the following account of an outbreak of disease 'similar to the Black Death', according to Gasquet, which appeared in the *British Medical Journal* of 5 November 1892. This account quotes an official report of the Governor General of Turkestan, published in St Petersburg, stating that the province had recently suffered an epidemic of the Black Death. On 10 September it appeared suddenly at Askabad and in six days killed 1303 out of a population of 30,000. The preface to the actual account of the disease said: 'Black Death has long been known in Western Asia as a scourge more deadly than the cholera *or the plague*'. This disease was, then, considered to be a separate disease from plague. It was then described and I quote from the original account in full:

> It comes suddenly, sweeping over a whole district like a pestilential simoon, *striking down animals as well as men*, (my italics) and vanishes as suddenly as it

came, before there is time to ascertain its nature or its mode of diffusion. The visit here referred to was no exception to this rule. After raging in Askabad for six days the epidemic ceased, leaving no trace of its presence but the corpses of its victims. These putrefied so rapidly that no proper post-mortem could be made.

The attack begins with rigors of intense severity, the patient shivering literally from head to foot; the rigors occur every five minutes for about an hour. Next an unendurable feeling of heat is complained of; the arteries become tense, and the pulse more and more rapid, while the temperature steadily rises. Unfortunately no thermometric readings or other precise data are given. Neither diarrhoea nor vomiting has been observed. Convulsions alternate with syncopal attacks, and the patients suffer intense pain. Suddenly the extremities become stiff and cold, and in from ten to twenty minutes the patient sinks into a comatose condition, which speedily ends in death. Immediately after he has ceased to breathe large black bullae form on the body, and quickly spread over its surface. Decomposition takes place in a few minutes.

It is not clear from this description how long the disease took from start to finish. One point of note is the comment that it struck down animals as well as men. This disease has little obvious similarity to bubonic plague, was clearly seen as a separate entity, and I can find no attempt to identify it in the literature. It seems curious, too, that Gasquet should have considered it to be so similar to the Black Death. It is worth noting, though, that Gasquet, in giving details of the 1348–9 epidemic, states that, 'some were struck suddenly and died within a few hours: others fell into a deep sleep, from which they could not be roused; whilst others, again, were racked with a sleepless fever, and tormented with a raging thirst'.

At Constantinople the Emperor John Cantacuzene, an eye witness of what he reported, described the epidemic which raged in northern Scythia in 1347 and spread widely throughout the Mediterranean. This was the disease which is held to be the Black Death. According to Gasquet the Emperor wrote that the course of the disease varied; some died suddenly, others during the course of a day, and some after only an hour's suffering. In the case of those lingering two or three days the attack commenced with violent fever. Soon the poison mounted to the brain and the sufferer lost the use of speech, became insensible to what was taking place about him and appeared sunk in deep sleep. If by chance he came to himself and tried to speak, his tongue refused to move and only a few inarticulate sounds could be uttered, as the nerves had been paralysed: then he died suddenly.

Others who fell sick under the disease were attacked first, not in the head, but in the lungs. These became quickly inflamed, sharp pains were experienced in the chest, blood was vomited and the breath became fetid. The throat and tongue, burnt up by the excessive fever, became black and congested with blood. Those who drank copiously experienced no more relief than those who drank but little. Finally, he described the terrible sleeplessness and restlessness of some sufferers and the plague spots which broke out over the body in most cases. This account in Gasquet makes no mention of buboes in groin or axilla.

According to Hecker (1859), Emperor John copied out some passages from Thucydides, 'though this was most probably only for the sake of rounding a period. This is no detriment to his credibility because his statements accord with the other accounts'. Bartsocas (1966) also draws attention to this feature and he usefully provides a verbatim account of the physical symptoms described by John.

Various versions provide a variety of information and it is extremely difficult to separate fact from myth in some. A few of the less lurid are worth consideration since points here and there deserve attention although in general we should not place too much reliance upon contemporary accounts of how the disease was transmitted. Boccaccio believed that the contagion was communicated not only by conversation with those who were sick but also by approaching them too closely, or even handling their clothes or anything they had previously touched. A Paduan chronicler noted that as a rule one sick man infected a house and that once the sickness entered a dwelling all were infected, *even the animals*. An anonymous Italian writer (in Gasquet) said the sickness was a 'swift and sharp fever, with blood-spitting, carbuncle or fistula'. Infection, he thought, was by talking to people but in the following account he clearly gave little importance to the blood contact: 'And here I can give my testimony. A certain man bled me, and the blood flowing touched his face. On that same day he was taken ill, and the next he died; and by the mercy of God I have escaped'. Of course the man who died may have already been incubating the disease. This writer said that the disease went on from February till 1 November 1348.

At Montpellier, a doctor called Simon de Covino called the disease 'pestis inguinaria', or bubonic plague of the East. He described it as having a burning pain, beginning under the arms or in the groin and extending to regions of the heart. A mortal fever then spread to the vital parts; the heart, lungs and breathing passages being chiefly affected. This account seems at variance with *bubonic* plague for once the buboes have appeared there is little likelihood of the disease then involving the respiratory system as he indicates and as it would in *pneumonic* plague alone, which would be unlikely to show buboes. This doctor observed that the disease progressed in hot or cold weather, spreading during the colder season of winter as rapidly as in the heat of the summer months and being found in high and healthy situations as well as in damp, low places. He was convinced that it was *contagious* by touch or breath and that mortality was greatest among the poor. He mentioned the fact that the animals such as dogs, cats, cocks and hens also died but whether of the disease or the lack of attention when their owners died was not clear.

Gui de Chauliac, a medical attendant of Pope Clement VI said the plague began in January 1348 and lasted for seven months. During the first two months the disease consisted mainly of constant fever and blood spitting of which the sick died in three days. For the next five months, in addition to constant fever, there were external carbuncles, or buboes, under the arm or in the groin and this ran its course in five days. He observed that the contagion was so great, especially when there was blood spitting, that not only by remaining with the sick but even by looking at them people seemed to take it. This account at any rate has some likeness to true plague. Yet what is believed to be this same disease behaved differently farther north, as a Bruges cleric wrote, 'for in Burgundy, Normandy and elsewhere it has consumed, and is consuming, many thousands of *men, animals and sheep*', and in Tournay it was said that in many houses the dogs and even cats died. Here, though, the disease was particularly severe among the chief people and the rich.

Hecker (1859) was of the opinion that on account of the inflammatory boils and the black spots indicative of a putrid decomposition, which appeared upon the skin, the disease was called the Black Death in Germany and the northern kingdoms of Europe. His account of the records of Emperor John Cantacuzene gives more details than that of Gasquet. He says that the Emperor noticed great imposthumes of the thighs and arms and comments that these indicate buboes, 'the infallible signs of the oriental plague', for he also mentioned separate smaller boils on arms, face and other parts of the body and distinguished these from the blisters also produced in plague. In addition he says that *black spots* broke out all over the body, either single or united and confluent. Unfortunately, I can find no mention of whether these were the skin haemorrhages beneath the surface or whether they were spots raised above the surface. The fauces and tongue were black and as if suffused with blood.

In the West, however, Hecker gives a series of symptoms which differ in some important respects from the disease in the region of Constantinople, the following being the predominating symptoms: an ardent fever, accompanied by *an evacuation of blood*, proved fatal in the first three days. He goes on to report that buboes and inflammatory boils did not at first come out at all but that the disease, 'in the form of carbuncular (anthrax-artigen) affection of the lungs, effected the destruction of life before the other symptoms were developed'.

In this form plague occurred in Avignon for a couple of months or so and then a disease with buboes in axilla and groin and with inflammatory boils all over the body made its appearance. This disease in Avignon first appeared in 1348 and lasted from January to August. The second episode was 12 years later in the autumn when it was reputed to have returned from Germany and raged for nine months. It would be odd for it to flare up in the autumn and go through the winter; furthermore, nine months would be a long time for epidemic plague to persist in one town. On its first appearance this disease raged chiefly among the poor but in 1360 it was more prevalent amongst the upper classes. In the second bout, children suffered severely, unlike 1348, but few women did so.

Hecker's account shows further variations in the disease in various parts of Europe. In Florence there were tumours in groin and axilla as large as an apple or egg, as well as other tumours all over the body, together with black or blue spots on arms, thighs or other parts. Although most died within the first three days after these symptoms appeared, there was generally no fever; as Hecker says, this was a very unusual circumstance in plague epidemics.

Michael of Piazza (Michael Platiensis) described the disease when it arrived in Sicily (in Nohl, 1926). He said that the arrivals bore in their bones a disease so virulent that even those who only spoke to them contracted the infection which was invariably fatal, the disease spreading to all who had any intercourse with the infected. Those who became infected had a severe pain throughout their bodies and then there developed on their thighs or upper arms a boil about the size of a lentil which the people called 'burn boil' (antrachi). This so infected the body that the patient violently vomited blood, such vomiting lasting without pause for three days at the end of which time, there being no means of healing it, the patient died. Other folk who contacted them died and even those who touched or used any things belonging to the diseased also suffered the same fate.

In Catania, where all died, there developed not only the 'burn blisters' but what are called gland boils. These were found on the sexual organs in some and on thighs, arms and the neck in others. These lesions were at first as large as a hazel nut and their development was accompanied by violent shivering so that those infected were too weak to stand and had to take to their beds where they had a violent fever. The boils grew to reach the size of a hen or a goose egg and were very painful and irritated the body, causing it to vomit blood. This account also states that the blood arose from the affected lungs to the throat so that we may not be really sure whether true vomiting did take place.

In Germany, because different reports gave different symptoms, Hecker concluded that the reporting was inaccurate. It may have been, but he did not apparently consider the alternative, namely that the chroniclers were recording different diseases. The mortality was not so great as in the other parts of Europe. Hecker was puzzled because not all the German accounts mention blood spitting, a feature which he considered diagnostic. Where it was mentioned, Hecker regarded the account as dubious because the deaths of those affected did not take place until the sixth or eighth day, an especially long interval because no other writers presented anything like so long a period. As we know from modern epidemics of pneumonic plague, it would be a very long time indeed, especially as plague was thought to be contacting the populace for the first time. The important point about this is, of course, the attitude of Hecker and the fact that, having plague fixed in his mind as the cause of the heavy mortality, all other diseases were ignored and their chroniclers treated as inaccurate.

In Norway 'the plague broke out in its most frightful form, with *vomiting of blood*' (Hecker, 1859). If this is accurate and it is certain that the difference between spitting blood and vomiting blood was known, then this might be a quite different disease pattern from the other forms described elsewhere.

In England the vomiting of blood is again referred to by Hecker. He says that the disease appeared, as at Avignon, with blood spitting and the same mortality, so that those who either manifested this symptom or with *vomiting of blood* either died immediately, within twelve hours or two days at the latest. Boils and buboes were also seen. In the British Isles, Gasquet claimed that in Ireland many died from abscesses, imposthumes and pustules on thighs and under the armpits, and whilst others died from affection of the head, as if in a frenzy, others died through *vomiting of blood*.

According to Hecker, only two *medical* descriptions of the epidemic have reached us. These were the accounts of Gui de Chauliac, who described the blood spitting and the buboes in some detail, and Raymond Chalin de Vinario, who observed blood coughing and in addition epistaxis (bleeding from the nose), hematuria (blood in the urine or bleeding from the urinary organs) and fluxes of blood from the bowels. Patients presenting these symptoms usually died on the same or the following day. None of these latter three features are characteristic of plague but may provide useful evidence of another disease. It would appear that Hecker's researches led him to believe that blood vomiting was common when he says that 'a vomiting of blood may not, here and there, have taken place'. Although he talks a lot about this phenomenon he does point out the difficulty of distinguishing a flow of blood from the stomach from a pulmonic expectoration.

The physician Chalin witnessed the epidemic of 1348 and the plagues of 1360, 1373 and 1382, and described affections of the throat which occurred in few cases and consisted of carbuncular inflammation of the gullet which caused difficulty in swallowing and even suffocated the patient in addition to which, in some instances, was added inflammation of the ceruminous glands of the ears, with tumours producing great deformity. Such patients, as well as others, coughed blood but as a rule they did not die before day six and even as late as day 14. Hecker goes on to point out – but does not elaborate – that a similar occurrence was often seen in other pestilences, as were also blisters on the body near which tumid glands and boils surrounded by discoloured and black streaks develop. He considered that these indicated the reception of the poison. The name given to these streaked spots was the girdle.

Plague eruptions were described as being *exanthemata viridia* (greenish boils, like a sea anemone), *caerulea* (blue), *nigra rubra* (black and red as a bruise), *lata* (broad), *diffusa* (spread out, a rash) and *velut signata punctis* (a puncture-like mark). Gasquet talks of small black pustules distributed over the whole skin of the body. He fails to elaborate on this but by his explicit use of the term one must assume that he distinguishes from petechiae. Shrewsbury, too, draws attention to these and also to other features. The plague-infected were, according to the account from Galfridi le Baker, 'afflicted by swellings which appeared suddenly in various parts of the body, which were so hard and dry that when lanced hardly any fluid came from them; many people recovered from these by lancing or long endurance. Others had small black blisters scattered over the whole body; from which very few, I might almost say hardly any, recovered to life and health'. Shrewsbury averred that these buboes were homologous with those described by Dioscorides and Posidonius.

Creighton (1894) indicates that the Black Death showed at least one important difference from later epidemics when he says, 'It is this universality of incidence that chiefly distinguishes the Black Death from the later outbreaks of plague, which were more often in towns than in villages or scattered houses, and were seldom in many places in the same year'.

Shrewsbury (1971), discussing the term Black Death, says that death from plague is no blacker than from any other microbial disease and whilst the corpse may show a purplish discolouration it does not turn black. He considers that smallpox has a better claim to the title and cites the Milan smallpox epidemic of 1888 where the corpses of some fulminant cases at Salerno had a charred appearance. An epidemic of cholera in Egypt was termed a 'black death' and in fatal cases he says that the extremities and the face and neck assume a slate-blue colouration as a result of the stagnation of the circulation in cutaneous blood-vessels. MacArthur (1926) can offer no explanation of how the fourteenth-century epidemic came to be called the Black Death but, perhaps significantly, he says that, 'the usual explanation that it was so called from the frequency of *vomiting of black blood* is not very convincing'.

Smallpox is another disease producing symptoms which affect the skin in a variety of ways. The virus usually infects via the upper respiratory tract, passing to the reticuloendothelial[18] cells where it multiplies and goes to the blood stream. It is carried to the skin and mucous membranes where the lesions are produced. In the skin, pustules are formed which, as healing begins and the contents dry up, form a thick crust of dead epithelial cells. In haemorrhagic smallpox there is an intense erythema[18] and purpuric spots of *purpura variolosa* casued by haemorrhages into the corium.[18] This is absent in the ordinary pustule. The rash may spread until the whole body is covered with large confluent areas of purpura. In addition to the skin haemorrhages, the patient may bleed from every body orifice. The fauces[19] may be black with submucosal bleeding and blood may pour from nose or mouth. Haemoptysis[19] may occur from bleeding into the alveoli,[19] bronchi or trachea. Haematemesis[19] or melaena[19] from bleeding into the gastro-intestinal tract can be evident and haematuria[19] and uterine haemorrhages may be present.

There is no hard roof to the vesicles in the mucous membranes (because they lack a hard epidermal layer) and the pharynx has an ulcerated appearance. The onset of smallpox is characterised by malaise, restlessness and severe headache. The temperature rises and the patient experiences chilliness and rigors with backache. Sleeplessness is evident, delirium is common and maniacal symptoms are occasionally present (Christie, 1980).

Patients are more infectious in the early stages of the eruptive phase. Ulcers in the mucous membrane break down and release virus to the air passages and out to the air. Later in the disease the skin is infectious. Christie is of the opinion that general widespread aerial convection of smallpox virus is unlikely and that fairly close human presence is necessary.

Whilst bubonic plague and smallpox all produce marked, dark skin rashes, they are not alone in doing so and several other diseases produce similar effects. In typhus (Christie, 1980) the rash often becomes a true petechiae and may darken along with the development of gangrene in the extremities. As the patient dies the skin turns mottled. During the English Civil War this appearance was called, 'an over-spreading of Blackness over the whole body' (MacArthur, 1959). A similar characteristic was recorded in the Turkestan disease mentioned earlier but typhus, unlike that disease or plague, goes on into the third week when, if the patient is to recover, the fever leaves him. During the initial febrile stage of relapsing fever there is bronchitis and transitory purpurae or erythematous eruptions are common on the neck, shoulder girdle, abdomen ands chest. Carried by the body louse, this disease was probably unlikely to be confused with plague because it is characterised by febrile periods lasting for two to ten days alternating with fever-free periods of two to four days. The overall mortality is given as two to ten per cent but in one closely observed epidemic in West Africa it was as high as 75 per cent (Imperato, 1974). It is not stated precisely but one assumes that this means the case mortality.

Typhoid fever produces the characteristic rose spots after one week of rising temperature and malaise. Often there are only four or five spots, 20 would be profuse in this disease. Because of the small number of rose spots in typhoid fever, it is tempting to think that the seventeenth-century accounts of patients with the plague 'spot' might be describing typhoid fever rather than bubonic plague.

In the worst cases of pharyngeal diphtheria there may be skin haemorrhages and bleeding from the nose and mouth. The infection of the faucial mucous membrane is accompanied by enlargement of the lymph nodes of the neck. This is often severe but as the whole neck is swollen it may be difficult to feel the separate nodes. Many writers on plague have drawn attention to the fetid breath of the victims. Diphtheria forms a coagulum in the throat and nasopharynx and the breath of such patients has a foul smell but, as Christie points out, any necrotic exudate will produce the same odour so that this feature cannot be considered unique to plague, nor even to diphtheria.

Organisms closely related to *Yersinia pestis* are responsible for disease in domestic and wild animals as well as man and should be considered in any attempt at analysing past epidemics. Tularaemia, a disease of wild rodents and man, is caused by the bacterium *Yersinia tularensis* which produces a disease in wild rodents with lesions resembling those in true plague-infected animals. In countries where plague exists, this infection has to be considered in the diagnosis of plague. Tularaemia is found in the western states of America, Japan, U.S.S.R., Yugoslavia, Norway and certain other parts of Europe (Cruickshank, 1965). Man becomes infected through handling infected animals and the disease is also spread by ticks and other biting arthropods. It may also be water-borne and according to Cruickshank water-rats may be infected and contaminate water by their excreta. Whether he means the common rat (*Rattus norvegicus*) which may live alongside water courses, or the more aquatic water vole (*Arvicola amphibius*), incorrectly called the water-rat, is not known. In man there may be ulcers of the skin and swelling of lymph nodes with a prolonged febrile illness. Before antibiotics, 9.5 per cent of recorded cases of tularaemia were fatal, a not inconsiderable mortality.

Other organisms of the *Yersinia* group have been responsible for important epizootic and enzootic disease in domesticated and wild animals but whilst they may infect man, such cases are infrequent today. *Y. multocida* (= *Y. septica*) has a world-wide distribution in animals: it causes a haemorrhagic septicaemia known variously as transit fever or stockyard disease in cattle, pneumonia with septicaemia in pigs, known as swine plague, and fowl cholera and septicaemia in poultry. Cases of human infection occur, especially in septic wounds following cat or dog bites.

Finally, *Yersinia pseudotuberculosis*, which occurs in a variety of wild rodents including *R. rattus* and *R. norvegicus* along with wood pigeons, can infect man but in modern times it appears that in the majority of cases human infections arise from domestic pets (Mair, 1968). In severe forms the disease in man is present as pseudotuberculous septicaemia which can be fatal.

It is remarkable how many bacterial and viral diseases produce skin rashes or petechiae, even diseases which primarily affect internal organs. Leptospirosis is a case in point where the spirochaete bacteria damage first of all the liver and later the kidneys. Petechiae, purpuric spots, may be present and skin rashes ranging from erythematous to urticarial. In addition there may be jaundice and severe bleeding from the alimentary or respiratory tract.

It is very likely that the people of the Middle Ages suffered from a wide variety of diseases. According to an Italian physician who wrote at the end of a medical career which encompassed the period from the 1650s to 1713, the health of peasants in the Campagna and the Po valley was miserable. They suffered from fever in summer, dysentery in the autumn and pleurisy and pneumonia in winter. At all seasons they regularly suffered from asthma, quinsy, erysipelas, digestive and intestinal ailments and bad teeth. D. Irsay (1927) says that during the thirteenth century there were distinguished twelve *morbi contagiosi* according to several authorities and these were probably: leprosy, influenza, trachoma, ophthalmic gonorrhea, scabies, impetigo, typhoid fever, anthrax, diphtheria, erysipelas, pulmonary tuberculosis and plague, to which could be added the deficiency disease of scurvy. This list does not mention smallpox or typhus and there may have been others, too.

An interesting piece of information relating to the fourteenth-century diseases is to be found in Leclainche (1936). He says, 'Dans la terrible épidémie de variole de 1345–50 (la mort noire, der Schwarze Tod), les chevaux, les moutons et les chèvres meurent par milliers'. Variole is smallpox (Latin variola) and not only did this great outbreak kill domestic animals but it was referred to as the *black death*. It also covered the period of the great mortality believed to be bubonic plague. This same writer gives some interesting information about earlier epidemics. Speaking of the great epidemic, 'qui désole la Gaule en 580, sous la règne de Childebert, et qui est mentionnée à la fois par dom Bouguet et par Grégoire de Tours', he says that this sickness spared not a single creature, all the herds of cattle were stricken and the deer died in the woods. Men in both town and countryside died at this time. In 791 the horses in Charlemagne's army had a severe disease which destroyed 90 per cent of them. In 801 there was plague in Charlemagne's empire which took men and animals alike and in 840 there was plague in men and horses. Between 810 and 1316 there were epizootics in cattle and horses.

Several other writers have commented that concurrent with human disease there was a heavy mortality amongst animals. In Gaza it was said that 22,000 people and most of the animals were carried off within six weeks but it is difficult to know how accurate was this estimate of human mortality. In Florence, 'as it advanced, not only men, but animals fell sick and shortly expired if they had touched things belonging to the diseased or dead'. It is said that Boccaccio saw two hogs snuffling about amongst the rags of a person who had died of plague and these animals, after staggering about for a short time, fell down dead, as if they had taken poison. It is difficult to evaluate this sort of record but he also says that multitudes of dogs, cats, fowls and other animals fell victims of the disease. Nicephoras Gregoras, a scholar and historian who wrote of the period 1204 to 1359, tells of a serious disease which not only destroyed men but animals living with and domesticated by man including dogs, horses, all the species of birds and 'even the rats that happened to live within the walls of the houses'. He says that prominent signs of the disease, indicating early death, were tumorous outgrowths at the roots of thighs and arms and bleeding ulcerations (in Bartsocas, 1966). If only rats had died along with men it would be better evidence of plague than a disease which was evidently catholic in its choice of species. Hecker says that the plague in England was soon accompanied by a fatal murrain among the cattle which, left without herdsmen, fell in their thousands. Rees (1923) says of the plague in London in 1348 that animals as well as men were affected 'but accurate evidence is not easily obtained'.

Around 1350 the monks of the Cathedral Priory of Christchurch requested the Bishop of Rochester to give them the church of Westerham to help them to maintain their traditional hospitality. They said that the great pestilence affecting man and beast made them unable to do this and claimed to have lost 257 oxen, 511 cows and 4585 sheep, worth in all £792–12–6d. According to Knighton the pestilence was succeeded by a murrain among domestic animals so that many sheep and oxen perished for lack of shelter and attention because of the dearth of serfs to look after them.

By 1350 the disease had reached Denmark and Schleswig Holstein where 'a great plague and sudden death raged both in the case of men and in that of cattle'. In 1369 the epidemic was described as a pestilence 'of men and the larger animals' (Thomas Walsingham).

It is unfortunate that few accounts of the fourteenth-century epidemic have been written by people who had expertise in medicine and it was not until 1568 that a treatise on plague in the British Isles appeared. This work, entitled *Ane Breve Description of the Pest*, was written by Gilbert Skeyne (1568) who, according to MacArthur (1926) was a professor of Medicine in the University of Aberdeen and physician to James VI of Scotland. MacArthur says that so far as he knows this was the first book published in this country by any physician dealing with plague and based on his own personal knowledge and observations, 'earlier writers having been content to translate from continental authors or to plagiarise from the ancients'. By this country MacArthur presumably means Britain: Shrewsbury says it was the first medical work on plague to be written in Scotland, perhaps implying that there had been even earlier ones in England although he does not go any further.

It seems extremely odd that this disease, which had been present for 220 years and which had been feared and blamed for so much, had not been written about by the medical profession from their first hand experience. As Creighton says, the reign of the plague in Britain was approaching an end before the native medical profession began to write about it. According to Skeyne, one of the signs of plague was when many animals died and he regarded it as an important indication of the onset of the disease when the 'Moudevart (= moudewarp or mole) and Serpent leavis the Eird (earth)'. However, Skeyne says so many curious things about the disease that these observations should perhaps be treated with caution.

With the exception of rodents there is little evidence that plague kills other mammals, even when infected experimentally. Simpson (1905) records that the German Plague Commission infected horses, oxen, sheep, goats, cats, dogs and pigs and of these only one goat died. The animals became ill and produced swellings at the point of infection but they recovered. However, experimentally infected monkeys died and so did rodents. Simpson comments that accounts of domestic and wild animals dying of plague seem to be indicative of something other than plague.

If, then, there is evidence of animal deaths at the time of plague, perhaps we ought to consider whether so-called plague in man might be related to animal disease. After all, many diseases are equally severe in man and domesticated species of animals, and any close spatial relationship of the two will facilitate rapid transmission of infectious or contagious disease. One of the most important shared diseases is anthrax, which is fatal to cattle, sheep, goats and horses, although swine are more resistant. Dogs and cats may become infected from eating the meat of anthrax victims and, whilst birds and fowls are said to be highly resistant, there have been outbreaks in ducks, geese and ostriches (Christie, 1980). The mortality in cattle, sheep and goats varies from 70–100 per cent and in horses is equally acute and fatal.

The name comes from the Greek word anthrax, meaning coal and from which we get the modern word anthracite. It also means a precious stone of dark-red colour, including the carbuncle, ruby and garnet, hence the carbuncle or malignant pustule which, according to some, refers to smallpox (Liddell and Scott, 1968). Because the centre of an anthrax pustule is jet black this is undoubtedly the reason for the English word anthrax and the French 'charbon' for this disease. According to Christie, the Anglo-Saxons called the disease the black bane. It was also probably the disease known as murrain in cattle. The *Anglo-Saxon Chronicle* (Garmonsway, 1955) mentions murrains along with plague, for example in A.D. 897: 'The host, by the mercy of God, had not altogether crushed the English people; but they were much more severely crushed during those three years by murrain and plague'. In A.D. 986 it was said that 'the great pestilence among cattle came first to England' but it is not known whether this was an entirely new disease or the recrudescence of one that had not been in evidence for some time. Human disease, 'plague', was often severe and in the year A.D. 995 there is a comment which could have come straight from the fourteenth century: 'there was so severe a plague that no more than five monks were left in Christ Church'. Pestilence was recorded in the *Chronicle* during A.D. 661 and, interestingly, 'a great mortality of birds' in the year A.D. 671.

The anthrax bacillus is a much hardier and more versatile organism than is *Yersinia pestis*. It can live outside the body of a vertebrate animal for long periods and remain infective, and is not dependent upon the biological vagaries of other species of animals as vectors. In the blood of an animal dying of anthrax or in a local pustule the anthrax bacilli are present in great numbers. It is common for dark, black blood to be voided from any of the natural body orifices and this blood will contain large numbers of the vegetative forms and hence be highly infective. When an animal dies of anthrax the survival and spread of the bacilli will depend to a great extent on the external temperature and whether the body is opened or not. If the carcass is left to lie unopened at a temperature of 28–30°C no bacilli will be recovered from the body after 80 hours because the anthrax bacilli find it difficult to compete with the organisms of putrefaction, which overwhelm them. At a lower temperature of 5–10°C putrefaction is less marked because the organisms are inhibited and vegetative anthrax bacilli may be found in the carcass after three or four weeks.

Spores form only in the presence of oxygen. The absence of calcium chloride enhances sporulation whilst its presence inhibits spore forming, thus spore formation and persistence might vary in different soils. A temperature of 20°C or less slows down spore formation when bacilli are freed from a carcass and other soil organisms may overcome them before they can sporulate. At higher temperatures they rapidly form spores and then their survival is certain. The spores are highly resistant to all agents and survive for long periods. Under experimental conditions on dried blood swabs or in paper envelopes they have survived for up to 68 years. In one experiment *B. anthracis* stored in dry soil survived for 60 years although the position is not clear in natural soil because of the effects of moisture, temperature and competition from other organisms.

When anthrax bacilli contact man the result will be either a severe cutaneous manifestation or involve lungs and intestines. Today, the introduction of antibiotics has reduced the death rate from cutaneous anthrax to a very low level but visceral anthrax is little affected by antibiotic treatment and the death rate may be as high as 90 per cent.

The incubation period is probably two to three days but may be shorter in pulmonary anthrax. Lesions begin as small pimples (papules) a few millimetres across, sometimes with a tiny vesicle on top. On the second day a ring of tiny vesicles appears surrounding the central papule. These are initially clear but as they enlarge take on a bluish colour, the contents becoming dark or blood stained. The central papule ulcerates and dries to form a dark brown depressed scab which during the next day or two turns black and as the surrounding vesicles dry up the scab enlarges to cover them so that by day five the lesion consists of a thick black scar. When fully developed the lesions may be three-quarters to one inch in diameter, but many are half this size, and a large one may measure two to three inches across. These measurements only refer to the sore itself, the accompanying tissue swelling may spread yet further. Inflammation of associated lymph nodes is frequent and these may be as large as a walnut and tender to the touch.

The general symptoms accompanying the cutaneous lesions are those of considerable upset, chilliness being the most common symptom along with headache, lack of appetite and nausea. In severe cases rigors may be present with a high temperature in very severe cases. The presence of vomiting, weakness and a thready pulse are grave signs.

In pulmonary anthrax the onset is rapid. The patient feels sick and cold and may vomit or cough up blood and within an hour is acutely ill with difficulty in breathing, blueness of the skin and a high temperature. Sweating profusely, the patient is very frightened and axillary lymph nodes are palpable. Death takes place on the second or third day.

Writing in 1720 Dr Richard Mead presented a list of symptoms indicating infection with the plague. These are many and varied, some being common to many fevers, and it would be easy to single out enough to suit several cases. In this array he does, however, point out that in many patients blood flows from the nostrils, sometimes the stools and from bladder and mouth. He does not mention buboes in relation to the living but those who, after death, exhibited buboes, carbuncles or blotches were said to have died of the plague.

In modern times the disease has shown a high degree of virulence in animals. In 1945 one million out of fifteen million sheep in Iran died of anthrax and in 1947 over one million farm animals in Iran died from this disease. Unconfirmed reports from Russia (*New Scientist*, 1980)[20] speak of a high human mortality in an outbreak. According to Christie (1980) workers in goat-hair mills and similar places, exposed to high levels of spores, show a high degree of resistance to clinical infection but it is not known what degree of resistance exists among the general populace.

Murrain has been documented among domestic animals during the fourteenth century. In the Oxfordshire manor of Cuxham in 1334–5 it killed 58 sheep out of a flock of between 100 and 150. The manor formed part of Merton College estates and was used by the College as a place of refuge when plague was raging in Oxford but there is no reference to it being so used in the fourteenth century. The earliest mention was in 1509 when any member of the College who so wished might go to Cuxham to stay with the rector. In 1548 the farmer of the manor was obliged to receive the Fellows and Scholars whenever the Warden and senior members saw fit to send them, 'by reason of the plague or for other reasons'. During the plague epidemics of 1603 and 1625, arrangements were made for the whole College to retire to Cuxham (Harvey, 1965).[21]

Sabine (1933) says that the periods 1314–20 and 1346–89 were times of murrain among domestic animals and that whilst the first may have been confined to cattle, horses, sheep and pigs, the second spread among poultry and wild birds as well, with murrain among sparrows in 1366. The murrain of 1316 was severe on cows and sheep. During the second period there was murrain in the years 1346–9, 1363, 1369, 1370, 1385, 1386 and 1389.

On the manor of Heacham, Norfolk, there was murrain from 1346 to 1411 without pause and it attacked horses, cattle, sheep, pigs, chickens, ducks, geese, swans, pea-hens and even hives of bees (Harrod, 1867). There was probably more than one vertebrate disease, as well as an insect pathogen, at work here. As an example of the effect of the disease, 152 sheep and 190 lambs died in one year out of a total of around 733 sheep.

Unlike plague, which is found entirely in rodents, anthrax widely affects vertebrate animals and it has often been remarked upon that there was heavy mortality of farm and wild animals during the Middle Ages and earlier. Some of the reporting has an air of exaggeration about it such as that in Adamnan's *Life of Columba* where it is said that in A.D. 684 it was recorded in the Irish Annals that there was a mortality of all animals throughout the world for the space of three years and not one in a thousand escaped. This probably meant that there were extensive animal epidemics but the actual figures mean little.

There is an interesting comment in Gregory of Tours on the plague in France in around A.D. 590–1 which those writers who have taken the sixth-century series of epidemics to be bubonic plague have ignored: 'The plague is said not to have spared even the animals, and to have attacked both *cattle and deer.*' Nearer to the Great Pestilence are more precise references to animal deaths such as in Coulton (1930) where he writes of the year A.D. 1268, 'During the ravages of that cattle-plague which men call Lungessouth in London this year'. It is interesting that as late as 1865 the term cattle-plague was still in use, this time it referred to rinderpest (Prothero, 1919).

The symptoms concerning animals in the fourteenth century are even less well recorded than those of men and it would be a gross oversimplification to suggest that anthrax was the only, or even the chief, animal disease of the times. It is, though, probably equally fatal to man and this, coupled with its symptoms and its high mortality rates, means that it must be a prime contender for the alternative position. Furthermore, it needs no vectors, the spores being the agent of infection and easily carried in the air or on skins, furs and wool and it is for this reason that anthrax has been known as 'wool sorters disease'.

This was the age of wool (Power, 1941; Lloyd, 1977) and Pelham (1951) reckons that in the mid-fourteenth century there was a total of 8,000,000 sheep in England. These, he says, were found in the lowland regions generally with the marshlands in particular supporting large numbers in spite of the diseases which were prevalent, although he unfortunately fails to elaborate on these diseases. The main concentrations were on the South Downs, especially to the east and many were found around Chichester on the parishes of the coastal plain. In Yorkshire and Lincolnshire the Cistercian abbeys had large flocks: Fountains Abbey had 15,000 and Rievaulx 12,000.

The effect of the Great Pestilence was seen in the price of wool, which fell from 1s–10⅝d per 7lb clove in 1347 to 1s–5d in 1348 and 1s–0d in 1349, probably because of the fall in the continental demand (Rogers, 1866). (The index of wool prices has been criticised, not least by Rogers himself.) He makes mention of murrain and points out that the losses to the medieval farmer were enormous as a result of this. In the year 1333 the following examples of sheep mortality due to murrain are given:

Maldon	– more than 50 per cent of sheep and lambs lost
Letherhead	– almost 50 per cent loss
Farley	– more than 25 per cent
Wolford & Basingstoke	– around 34 per cent
Wolford	– below 14 per cent
Cuxham	– around 11 per cent

Rogers says that similarly heavy losses can be found in other years.

Not only sheep but cattle also were plentiful and widespread (Donkin, 1962–3). Attempts to assess numbers are difficult but Postan (1962–3) showed the probable numbers of sheep, horses and cattle in south Wiltshire in 1225. The average holding of animals per taxpayer was: sheep – 15.6; horses and cattle – about 2.5 but such figures varied from region to region. As in the case of sheep, the Cistercian monasteries held large herds of cattle (Donkin, 1962–3).

Murrains had clearly been recorded on many occasions before 1348 in sheep and cattle (Kershaw, 1973) and the term covered a variety of diseases in much the same way as the term plague did in men. The genesis of animal diseases and especially their identification is a very difficult task for the period in question. It is an intriguing point that in some instances there may have been a move of disease from wild animals to domesticated species for Kershaw points out that of the nine murrains mentioned in the chronicles between A.D. 1086 and 1283, the first three, in 1086, 1103 and 1111, were called mortality of animals whereas the outbreak of A.D. 1131 was a mortality of domestic animals and those of 1201, 1225, 1258, 1277 and 1283 were murrains largely affecting sheep. Murrains carried on throughout the centuries and in 1538 destroyed one seventh of the flock of Tavistock Abbey. Sheep scab was clearly known because the Abbey records show the purchase of tar and tallow (Finberg, 1951).

Although recorded on many occasions before 1348, murrains had never been accompanied by such an unprecedented human epidemic and this leads me to think that the Great Pestilence was caused by an organism not only common to man and animals but, because of its severity, perhaps new to both of them. The clinical symptoms in man strongly suggest anthrax more than any other disease known today and the supporting evidence against bubonic plague leads me to the conclusion that northern Europe may have been experiencing its first exposure to anthrax.

The route by which plague is reputed to have reached Europe could be the very same one that anthrax used. Ennen (1979) says that between 1204 and 1261 there is mention of a special quarter of Constantinople which belonged to the merchants of the south of France. This was under Venetian authority but, from the early thirteenth century, control of trade between southern France and North Africa decreased and direct trade between Marseilles and the Saracens boomed. Arles, Saint-Gilles, Montpellier and Marseilles were involved in this trade and the chief imports of Marseilles were skins, furs, wool and some other commodities and presumably these found their way northwards in the trading process.

In thirteenth-century Europe there was a well-organised trade in pelts and manufactured furs. The Paris sales of skins and furs were renowned and Marseilles merchants collected skins from Spain, Sicily and North Africa. By the late thirteenth century, Bruges was becoming the centre for western Europe, a position it held for the next 200 years, and at that time skins from the northern countries as well as the Iberian peninsula and Fez, Tunis, 'Sardinia and Tatary, beyond the shores of the Black Sea' (Veale, 1966).

If anthrax had come from the East it could have been swiftly spread across Europe from Marseilles and other ports. In north-western Europe there were some 150 cloth towns, 90 of them in the Low Countries, and they exported to the Mediterranean and also by way of the German Hanse to the Baltic and presumably received hides and wool from southern France. Genoa, prominent in plague folk-lore, was a cloth transit centre and Ennen says that the city obtained cloths from the northern cities via the Rhône valley and despatched them either from its harbour for export by ships or over the Alps and through Piedmont.

The cloth industry was the main feature of the economy of the urban area between the Seine and the Rhine and there was a dense aggregation of smaller cloth settlements around Ypres, a cloth town where famine had reputedly been so severe. One may speculate that hand in hand with famine there may have been a history of disease associated with the wool trade for many years before the epidemic of 1347–50.

In a climatic zone like northern Europe where the Black rat, if it existed at all, would be confined to the warmest quarters of ports and towns, plague could not have been expected to be, as it was supposed to be in the fourteenth century, a disease of villages and countryside. A disease like anthrax, with a simpler spreading mechanism would, once established, be present in the soil for many years ahead. It is known today that deep ploughing will disturb old anthrax graves and this has happened on the Berkshire Downs near East Ilsley (A. McDiarmid, pers. comm.), a sheep fair centre where sheep probably died and were either not buried at all or put in shallow graves. There are in many areas 'anthrax fields' where cattle are not kept and only shallow cultivation is carried out for fear of disturbing the spores of anthrax. Even these precautions may be in vain because soil invertebrates, particularly earthworms, will bring spores to the surface.

The high infectivity of the Great Pestilence has always been a feature of contemporary comment. Thucydides' account of the plague of Athens said, 'Appalling too was the rapidity with which men caught the infection; dying like sheep if they attended one another; and this was the principal cause of mortality'. Similar sentiments were frequently expressed during the fourteenth century. It is also worth noting that people had a great dread of the corpses of so-called plague victims, a fear which has no basis in fact in bubonic plague but is highly relevant in cases of anthrax. It is of course possible that the same unreasoning fear would have been present in the case of any new disease since people had no understanding of the mechanisms of disease transmission.

According to Wood (1865) plague reached London in December 1664 in woollen goods from Holland and arrived in Eyam in materials sent to a tailor. Certainly anthrax would seem a more appropriate disease in the Peak village of Eyam than would bubonic plague. Another point, too, is worth mentioning in connection with the Eyam epidemic. The people of the village were prevented or dissuaded from leaving the village, as a result of which the death rate was high and it is said that this martyrdom prevented the disease from spreading beyond the parish. This may equally be evidence of a disease which was either contagious or infectious from person to person. The high mortality of the Eyam epidemic is interesting in the light of an observation by Galfridi le Baker who spoke of a peculiarly fatal form, from which few or none recovered; it was characterised by small black pustules on the skin. This was during the 1348–50 epidemic but even then the skin eruptions were noticed at a time when there was probably a wide variety of abscesses, rashes and blemishes.

It is said that George Vicars, the first person to die in Eyam, became ill soon after opening the box of clothes from London. He may well have done so but we have no proof that he contracted his illness *from* the clothes and he may have already been incubating the disease when he opened the box. The assumption that he became infected from the contents of the box has raised problems for those attempting to fit plague to this situation. The short incubation period would virtually rule out bubonic plague and the fact that he had buboes eliminates both pneumonic and septicaemic forms. Pneumonic plague can be further discounted because the next case did not occur for another two weeks. The suggestion that a human flea, brought in earlier by a visitor to Eyam Wakes on 20 August, 13 or 14 days before Vicars became ill, is unlikely because such a vector would be more likely to have been passed direct to Vicars and his illness would have begun earlier than it did. Furthermore, the human flea is a poor plague carrier, even when plague is present. The 'plague spot' appeared on George Vicars' breast and perhaps, as I have said earlier, we should seriously consider typhoid in this instance.

Some observations made concerning the distribution of plague mortality in the Black Death and which appeared difficult to reconcile with bubonic plague might make more sense if we postulate anthrax in a country with a very high population of sheep. Shrewsbury (1971) points out that Lunn confessed to being puzzled by the fact that the most mountainous deanery in the diocese of Bath and Wells, that of Dunster, had the greatest number of vacant benefices, saying, 'In the recesses of Exmoor itself there were few parishes which escaped – Dulverton, Winsford, Exford, Cutcombe, Stoke Pero, Porlock and Culbone form one unbroken chain of parishes which saw a change of parson in the plague'. Shrewsbury complains that Lunn's siting of the parishes is at fault, only Stoke Pero and Exford being within Exmoor, the rest lying on the fringes of the moor and being accessible during the summer from Porlock Bay or Minehead and Watchet. Dulverton, however, is on the southern edge of Exmoor, in a deep valley whose drainage runs south. Perhaps more to the point is the fact that Exmoor was then, as today, a major sheep rearing and grazing area. Shrewsbury thinks that plague would have radiated inland wherever rats were present in sufficient density to support epizootics of plague. He believes that the wool trade would have assisted the rat to colonise the five fringe hamlets but doubts whether by 1348 it had penetrated to Exford and Stoke Pero in sufficient numbers to sponsor epidemic plague. Dulverton is further from the northern ports and this makes the hypothesis even more untenable. However, if anthrax was the disease then all these parishes in this hilly deanery had a very close association with the wool trade in all its aspects and the difficulties associated with bubonic plague dissemination would be less of a problem. It is worth pointing out that the major period of the epidemic was from December to April in this diocese.

One final point remains to be mentioned and that is the question of the remarkable speed which the disease achieved in its passage northwards. Professor Colin Kaplan, with whom I discussed this matter, suggested that the rapid spread of the Great Pestilence pointed not merely to an inter-person aerosol transmission but to something still more swift and he drew my attention to current thinking on the spread of the virus which causes foot-and-mouth disease in livestock.

During 1967–8 the outbreaks of this disease in cattle and pigs in England led to studies on the airborne passage of the virus and the role of meteorological conditions in epidemics. An examination of the outbreaks in England during 30 years suggested that some, such as in 1952, were associated with favourable meteorological conditions at a key time for transport from the continent of Europe. Evidence showed that certain micro-organisms were widely available in fields on the Continent and present in considerable numbers at 10,000 feet over the North Sea (Hurst, 1968). Experimental work by Sellers and Parker (1969) into the airborne excretion of the virus showed that large amounts were excreted as an aerosol and these authors suggested that under conditions of relative humidity greater than 70 per cent and at low temperatures, survival of the virus to a distance of 100 kilometres was likely to occur.

In an outbreak of foot-and-mouth disease in Worcestershire in 1969 a study of climatic conditions and of the natural features of the area showed that the wind could have carried the virus from one or other of the three farms first infected to another 26 during the next two weeks (Henderson, 1969). Finally, Tinline (1970) suggested that the smooth air flow in lee waves could transport 'air parcels' along the streamline pattern of these waves and that such an air parcel could remain intact throughout its passage with the concentration of virus remaining similar to its concentration at its source of origin. Such an air parcel with a high virus concentration might come to ground level a long way downwind and the virus content could be deposited or inhaled at a high infective strength.

Ziegler (1970) has commented upon the patchy distribution of the Black Death in Cambridgeshire, where some manors lost many tenants whilst others not far away lost few, and remarks that no one has yet put forward any plausible suggestions to account for this. The airborne passage of parcels of bacteria in the manner outlined above might explain why there was this high local variation in death rates.

The extraordinarily rapid dissemination of the Black Death suggests pulmonary anthrax moving in a similar way. This form of the disease could very likely have been the illness which has hitherto been identified with pneumonic plague. Furthermore, it seems to me that the condition called 'malignant pustule' of the lung (p. 202) was probably pulmonary anthrax. Certainly, one of the definitions of anthrax as a splenic fever of sheep and cattle carries with it the added information that it causes malignant pustule in man when he becomes infected from animals but it does not make it clear whether this refers to external or internal lesions.

It is tempting to speculate yet further and to suggest that the sequence of earthquakes and floods in the East before the Black Death might have disturbed anthrax in the soil and the spores were then carried by air currents to the Mediterranean and Europe. Against this, though, is the fact that accounts of disease at Constantinople bear the stamp of true plague whereas those in Europe have less similarity.

Anthrax is widely known in African mammals, however, and air currents bearing spores of anthrax could easily reach northern Europe, as shown by the deposition of Saharan dust in England in recent years. Such a hypothesis would at any rate have a firmer basis in reality than that put forward by Professor Fred Hoyle who considered that the sporadic nature of plague outbreaks was due to the organisms coming in from outer space, the very small size of the particles and their low speed being sufficient to prevent them burning up on entry into the atmosphere. Speculation along these lines is unnecessary in the case of plague since the known biology of the disease can account for all the recorded epidemics. On theoretical grounds, though, it would be quite feasible for micro-organisms from some distant source, should one exist, to reach Earth in this way.

My main task has been to examine the Black Death from the viewpoint of the overall biology of the disease, integrating the characteristics of carriers with environment, medical symptoms and historical fact. Accounts of the medieval epidemic have concentrated mainly on the historical aspects and the biology has been largely overlooked, almost certainly because there has not been thought any need to question the long-held belief that it was plague. Yet, as I have attempted to show, plague and the Black Death have many discrepancies; too many for a comfortable acceptance that they are one and the same disease over most of the region in question. I have proposed a disease which can be considered as a leading alternative but it will have become obvious from the examples I have given that there are several diseases each of which have features fitting some of the events of the fourteenth century. This may be nearer the truth and it is likely that in addition to one main, new disease there was a spectrum of concurrent illnesses, deaths from which were likely to be attributed to the more spectacular arrival.

After the fourteenth century there were repeated outbreaks of disease called plague, yet even a superficial look at some of them is sufficient to raise doubts on this point. Perhaps we have blamed plague for too much and I hope that my views will encourage others to look again, not only at the Black Death but at the many later episodes of disease in the British Isles.

Notes to the text

1 (p. 15).   The title 'Plague Research Commission' is the name given to a body whose correct designation was 'The working Commission appointed by the Advisory Committee nominated by the Secretary of State for India, the Royal Society, and the Lister Institute of Preventive Medicine'.

The reports of the 'Commission' which was appointed in 1905 were published during the years 1906–17 under the title of 'Reports on Plague Investigations in India' in a series of special supplements and ordinary numbers of the *Journal of Hygiene*. Throughout this book, except where such reports are attributed to named authors, the reference will be 'Plague Research Commission' followed by the date.

2 (p. 18).   Ecchymoses are livid, and petechiae purple, spots in the skin due to blood which has escaped from nearby vessels.

3 (p. 47).   This version of the events at Caffa was largely based upon Haeser (H. Haeser, *Archiv für gesammte Medicin*, Jena, ii, 26–59) who in turn used the account of Gabriele de' Mussi. The latter's account of the Crimean incident was called *Ystoria de morbo seu mortalitate qui fuit a. 1348*. Haeser believed that de' Mussi was actually present at Caffa and returned to Europe in the plague ships. However, Tononi (A. G. Tononi, *'La Peste dell' Anno 1348'* published in *Giornale Ligustico*, Genoa, Vol. X, 1883) has shown that de' Mussi never left Piacenza at that time and must therefore have relied upon the accounts of others.

4 (p. 65).   I have been unable to read Dr Lunn's Ph.D. thesis because a copy was never deposited in the University Library (Board of Research Studies, 13 December 1950). My attempts at contacting Dr Lunn have also failed because I have been informed by the records office of St John's College, Cambridge that he was recorded as deceased in January, 1976. Furthermore, any hopes of getting in touch with his relatives have also been unavailing because the College no longer has an address for him.

5 (p. 75).   The long bones of limbs, hands and feet cease growth in length when the bony cap, the epiphysis, at each end of the long part, or shank, fuses with the shank.

This fusion represents the end of the growth period and is used as a point at which young may be separated from adults.

6 (p. 76). The *Muridae* comprise the rats and mice and the *Cricetidae* the voles amongst the Order of mammals called rodents. The *Muridae* have long tails relative to the length of head and body, e.g. *Rattus rattus*, and the *Cricetidae* have shorter tails, in some cases, such as the genus *Microtus*, much shorter than head-body length. The two groups may be also separated on tooth structure, which is very distinctive.

7 (p. 78). The bacterium responsible for bubonic plague was formerly called *Pasteurella pestis*. It has recently been reclassified and its name is now *Yersinia pestis*.

8 (p. 89). The embryo rate is a measure of the productivity of a species. It is the average number of embryos per pregnant female.

9 (p. 95). The legal area of deer forest jurisdiction may have covered a third of the country but this should not be confused with the area of actual woodland. The latter at the time of Domesday is thought to have covered about 13 per cent of the area of the survey.

10 (p. 98). Hallam (1957–8) used data from the Benedictine priory at Spalding to estimate the size of thirteenth-century peasant households. On the manor of Weston the size of households was 4.37, Moulton 4.72 and Spalding 4.81, all higher than the 3.5 per household calculated by Russell (1948).

11 (p. 126). Fleas, lice, mites and ticks live a parasitic existence on the outer body surface of vertebrate animals and are known as ectoparasites in contrast to endo-parasites which live internally. The latter include tapeworms, round worms and such organisms as the bacillus of *Yersinia pestis*.

12 (p. 128). The ingestion of invading micro-organisms by certain cells of the body which are specialised for this function is termed phagocytosis. The particular cells carrying out this activity in insects are called haemocytes and correspond to the macrophages of vertebrate animals.

13 (p. 151). *Salmonella* bacteria cause food poisoning in man and may be fatal to rodents. They were formerly used as rodent poisons but since much rodent control takes place near human food stores their use has for many years been banned.

14 (p. 169). To a biologist the word 'cline' means the gradation of form differences over a geographical area. The prefix 'patho' would imply a similar gradation in pathological organisms.

15 (p. 174). The degree of symmetry possessed by curves is quantified by the value β_1. If β_1 is small in value, e.g. 0.011, the curve is very nearly symmetrical and as the value of β_1 increases to, e.g. 0.806, the curve becomes more and more asymmetrical. Therefore, a series of values for β_1 referring to a series of epidemics thus describes roughly the degree of symmetry or asymmetry present in each case. For any perfectly symmetrical curve $\beta_1 = 0$.

The value β_2 describes the form of the curve. In the case of the normal curve of error, $\beta_2 = 3$ but as β_2 increases in value, e.g. 4.21, the curve becomes narrower and with a higher curvature at the apex than the normal curve. As β_2 falls towards 3, e.g. 3.15, the curve becomes broader and flatter at the apex.

16 (p. 195). It should be remembered that the decision to allow no one to leave the village and also to prevent anyone entering – though few would have wished to – meant that this became a closed community, a fact which may have resulted in a higher death rate.

17 (p. 198). For this translation I am indebted to Mr F. A. Wilford of the Department of Classics at Royal Holloway College. He is in no doubt that Robert of Avesbury meant more than 200 burials almost every day.

18 (p. 208).
Reticuloendothelial cells: mobile scavenging cells of the body
Erythema: irregularly defined red patches of the skin
Corium: the deeper layer of the skin

19 (p. 208).
Fauces: the back of the mouth, terminated by the pharynx and larynx
Haemoptysis: the coughing up of blood from the lungs
Alveoli: the air spaces in the lungs
Haematemesis: vomiting of blood from the stomach
Melaena: an intestinal evacuation mixed with altered blood, often black and
            sometimes like tar
Haematuria: the presence of blood in the urine

20 (p. 215). The United States State Department circulated a story that anthrax from a biological weapons establishment had infected many people with between 300 and 500 dead. The author of the article* points out that a severe outbreak of anthrax in Russia does not necessarily mean that the organisms had come from a biological weapons unit since there have been several well-documented natural outbreaks.

* *New Scientist*, 85, 1980 p. 986. Anthrax in the air.

21 (p. 215). There would have been little point in leaving Oxford for Cuxham during the Black Death since the epidemic was present there in the winter and early spring of 1349. Harvey (1965) considered that the population of the manor in 1377 was only one-third of its probable level in 1348 and that the immediate human mortality may have been even greater.

References

Chapter One

BACOT, A. W. & MARTIN, C. J., 'Observations on the mechanism of the transmission of plague by fleas', *Journal of Hygiene*, 13, 1914, pp. 423-39.

POLLITZER, R., *Plague. World Health Organization Monograph*, Series No. 22, Geneva, 1954.

SIMPSON, W. J., *A Treatise on Plague dealing with the Historical, Epidemiological, Clinical, Therapeutic and Preventive Aspects of the Disease*, Cambridge University Press, 1905.

CHUN, J. W. H., 'Clinical features', in WU, LIEN-TEH, CHUN, J. W. H., POLLITZER, R. & WU, C. Y., eds, *Plague, A Manual for Medical and Public Health Workers*, National Quarantine Service, Shanghai Station, China, 1936, pp. 309-33.

GILL, C. A., *The Genesis of Epidemics and the Natural History of Disease*, Baillière, Tindall & Cox, London, 1928.

SHREWSBURY, J. F. D., *A History of Bubonic Plague in the British Isles*, Cambridge University Press, 1971.

HANKIN, E. H., 'On the Epidemiology of Plague', *Journal of Hygiene*, 5, 1905, pp. 48-83.

TWIGG, G. I., 'The Role of Rodents in Plague Transmission: a worldwide review', *Mammal Review*, 8, 1978, pp. 77-110.

WU, LIEN-TEH, 'Historical aspects', in WU, LIEN-TEH, CHUN, J. W. H., POLLITZER, R. & WU, C. Y., eds, *Plague, A Manual for Medical and Public Health Workers*, National Quarantine Service, Shanghai Station, China, 1936, pp. 1-55.

SEAL, S. C., 'Epidemiological studies of plague in India. 2. The changing pattern of rodents and fleas in Calcutta and other cities', *Bulletin of the World Health Organization*, 23, 1969a, pp. 293-300.

SEAL, S. C., 'Epidemiological studies of plague in India. 1. The present position', *Bulletin of the World Health Organization*, 23, 1969b, pp. 283-292.

BANNERMAN, W. B., 'The Spread of Plague in India', *Journal of Hygiene*, 6, 1906, pp. 179–211.

HUTCHESON, G., 'Mahamari, or the Plague, in British Garhwal and Kumaon', *Transactions of the first Indian Medical Congress*, Calcutta, 1895, pp. 304–312.

THOMPSON, J. ASHBURTON, *Report on the outbreak of plague at Sydney, 1900*, Department of Public Health, New South Wales, 1900, pp. 1–49.

THOMPSON, J. ASHBURTON, 'On the epidemiology of plague', *Journal of Hygiene*, 6, 1906, pp. 537–69.

TIDSWELL, F., *Report on the outbreak of plague at Sydney, 1900*. Department of Public Health, New South Wales, Appendix A, Bacteriological Report, pp. 50–7.

MITCHELL, J. A., 'Plague in South Africa: historical summary', *Publications of the South African Institute for Medical Research*, 3, 1927, pp. 89–104.

ROBERTS, J. I., 'The Endemicity of Plague in East Africa', *East African Medical Journal*, 12, 1935, pp. 200–219.

Chapter Two

LATHAM, R. E., *Revised Medieval Latin Word List*, Oxford University Press, London, 1965.

SHREWSBURY, J. F. D., *A History of Bubonic Plague in the British Isles*, Cambridge University Press, 1971.

SHREWSBURY, J. F. D., *The Plague of the Philistines and other medical essays*, Victor Gollancz Ltd, London, 1964.

THUCYDIDES *Works*, translation by B. Jowett, Clarendon Press, Oxford, 1881.

MACARTHUR, W. P., 'The Medical Identification of some Pestilences of the Past', *Transactions of the Royal Society of Tropical Medicine and Hygiene*, 53, 1959, pp. 423–39.

PROCOPIUS, *History of the Wars*, Books I and II, translation by H. B. Dewing, Heinemann, London, 1914.

RUSSELL, J. C. 'That Earlier Plague', *Demography*, 5, 1968, pp. 174–184.

PIRENNE, H., *Mohammed and Charlemagne*, Unwin University Books, London, 1939.

GREGORY OF TOURS, *The History of the Franks*, (2 vols) translation by O. M. Dalton, Clarendon Press, Oxford, 1927, I, 421–2; II, 119, 141, 395, 516, 600.

McNEILL, W. H., *Plagues and Peoples*, Blackwell, Oxford, 1977.

DOLS, M. W., 'Plague in early Islamic Society', *Journal of the American Oriental Society*, 94, 1974, pp. 371–83.

BAUTIER, ROBERT-HENRI, *The Economic Development of Medieval Europe*, Thames and Hudson, London, 1971.

POLLITZER, R., *Plague, World Health Organization Monograph*, Series No. 22, Geneva, 1954.

BONSER, W., 'Epidemics during the Anglo-Saxon Period', *Journal of the British Archaeological Association*, 3rd series, 9, 1944, pp. 48–71.

LLOYD, Sir J. E., *A History of Wales. From the earliest times to the Edwardian conquest*, (2 vols), 3rd edn., London, Longmans, Green & Co, London, 1939, Vol. 1, p. 131.

The Anglo-Saxon Chronicle, translation by G. N. Garmonsway, J. M. Dent & Sons Ltd, London, 1955.

The Old English Version of Bede's Ecclesiastical History of the English people, edited and translated by Thomas Miller, published for the early English Text Society by N. Trübner and Co., London, 1890.

GEOFFREY of MONMOUTH, *The History of the Kings of Britain*, translated with an introduction by Lewis Thorpe, Penguin Books, 1966.

ADAMNAN (Saint), *The Life of Saint Columba (Columb-Kille)* A.D. 521–597, translation by Wentworth Huyshe, George Routledge & Sons, Limited, London, 1906.

Chapter Three

LANGER, W. L. 'The Black Death', *Scientific American*, 210, 1964, pp. 114–121.

PROCOPIUS *History of the Wars*, translation by H. B. Dewing, Heinemann, London, 1914, books I & II.

GREGORY OF TOURS, *The History of the Franks*, (2 vols) translation by O. M. Dalton, Clarendon Press, Oxford, 1927, I, 421–2; II, 119, 141, 395, 516, 600.

SHREWSBURY, J. F. D., *A History of Bubonic Plague in the British Isles*, Cambridge University Press, 1971.

McNEILL, W. H., *Plagues and Peoples*, Blackwell, Oxford, 1977.

MARINUS SANUTUS, *Liber secretorum Fidelium crucis super Terrae Sanctae recuperatione et conversatione*, in Bongars, *Gesta Dei per Francos*, vol. ii.

ZIEGLER, PHILIP, *The Black Death*, Pelican Books, England, 1970.

CHWOLSON, D., 'Syrisch-Nestorianische Grabinschriften Aus Semirjetschie', *Mémoires de l'Académie Impériale des Sciences de St.-Pétersbourg*, VII Serie, tome XXXVII, No. 8, 1890, p. 111, 113, 116, 131, 140.

STEWART, J., *Nestorian Missionary Enterprise. The story of a church on fire*, T. & T. Clark, Edinburgh, 1928.

POLLITZER, R., *Plague. World Health Organization Monograph*, Series No. 22, Geneva, 1954.

GASQUET, F. A., *The Black Death of 1348 and 1349*, George Bell and Sons, London, 1908.

MATTEO VILLANI, *Muratori, Rerum Italicarum Scriptores*, XIV, col. 14.

MATTEO VILLANI, *CRONICA ... con appendici storico-geografiche*, compilate da F. Gherardi-Dragomanni, 2 vols, Florence, 1846.

HECKER, J. F. C., *The Epidemics of the Middle Ages*, translated by B. G. Babington, 3rd edn., Trübner & Co., London, 1859.

STICKER, GEORG, *Die Pest. Abhandlungen aus der Seuchengeschichte und Seuchenlehre*, Bd. I. Giessen, 1908.

ALPINUS, PROSPER, *De Medicina Aegyptiorum*, Libiri Quatuor, Venetiis, 1591.

PETRIE, G. F. & TODD, R. E., 'A Report on Plague Investigations in Egypt', *Reports and Notes of the Public Health Laboratories, Cairo*, 5, 1923, pp. 1–114.

RUSSEL, PATRICK, *A Treatise of the Plague*, London, 1791.

AUBERT-ROCHE, L., *De la peste ou typhus d'Orient*, Paris, 1843.

GAETANI, FRANCESCO, *Sulla peste che afflisse l'Egitto l'anno 1835*, Naples, 1841.

VERNADSKY, G., *The Mongols and Russia*, Yale University Press, New Haven, 1953.

DE SMET, 'Breve Chronicon clerici ananymi', *Recueil des Chroniques de Flandres*, vol. III, p. 14.

MICHAEL OF PIAZZA (Platiensis), *Bibliotheca scriptorum qui res in Sicilia gestas retulere*, vol. I, p. 562.

BYRNE, E. J., *Genoese shipping in the twelfth and thirteenth centuries*, The Mediaeval Academy of America; Cambridge, Massachusetts, 1930.

PLINY, *Natural History*, translation by H. Rackham, William Heinemann Ltd., London, 1950, vol. V, book XIX, 1.

CREIGHTON, C., *A History of Epidemics in Britain*, 1894, 2nd edn., with additional material by D. E. C. EVERSLEY, E. A. UNDERWOOD, and L. OVENALL, Frank Cass & Co. Ltd, London 1965.

Chapter Four

CREIGHTON, C., *A History of Epidemics in Britain*, 1894, 2nd edn., with additional material by D. E. C. EVERSLEY, E. A. UNDERWOOD and L. OVENALL, Frank Cass & Co. Ltd, London 1965.

ZIEGLER, PHILIP, *The Black Death*, Pelican Books, England, 1970.

HANKIN, E. H., 'On the Epidemiology of Plague', *Journal of Hygiene*, 5, 1905, pp. 48–83.

BIRABEN, JEAN-NOËL, *Les hommes et la peste en France et dans les pays européens et méditerranéens*, tome I, *La peste dans l'histoire*, Mouton & Co. and Ecole des Hautes Etudes en Sciences Sociales, 1975.

LANGER, W. L., 'The Black Death', *Scientific American*, 210, 1964, pp. 114–121.

GASQUET, F. A., *The Black Death of 1348 and 1349*, George Bell and Sons, London, 1908.

ROBERTUS DE AVESBURY, *De Gestis Mirabilibus Regis Edwardi Tertii*, THOMPSON, EDWARD MAUNDE ed., H.M.S.O., 1889.

SHREWSBURY, J. F. D., *A History of Bubonic Plague in the British Isles*, Cambridge University Press, 1971.

BOUCHER, C. E., 'The Black Death in Bristol', *Transactions of the Bristol and Gloucestershire Archaeological Society*, Vol. LX, 1938, pp. 31–46.

THOMSON, EDWARD MAUNDE, ed., *Chronicon Galfridi le Baker de Swynebroke*, Clarendon Press, Oxford, 1889.

THOMPSON, A. HAMILTON, *The English Clergy and their Organization in the later Middle Ages*, Clarendon Press, Oxford, 1947.

FLETCHER, J. M. J., 'The Black Death in Dorset, (1348–1349)', *Dorset Natural History and Antiquarian Field Club*, Vol. XLIII, 1922, pp. 1–14.

HECKER, J. F. C., *The Epidemics of the Middle Ages*, translated by B. G. Babington, 3rd edn, Trübner & Co., London, 1859.

REES, W., 'The Black Death in Wales', *Transactions of the Royal Historical Society*, 4th series, vol. III, 1920, pp. 115–135.

RUSSELL, J. C., *British Medieval Population*, The University of New Mexico Press, Albuquerque, 1948.

PLAGUE RESEARCH COMMISSION, 'The epidemiological observations made by the Commission in Bombay City', *Journal of Hygiene*, 7, 1907, pp. 724–798.

PHILIP, W. M. & HIRST, L. F., 'A report on the outbreak of the plague in Colombo. 1914–1916', *Journal of Hygiene*, 15, 1917, pp. 527–564.

RUSSELL, J. C., 'That earlier plague', *Demography*, 5, 1968, pp. 174–184.

LUNN, J., *The Black Death in the Bishop's Registers*, Unpublished typescript copy of a thesis awarded the Ph.D. degree of Cambridge University, 1937.

THOMPSON, A. HAMILTON, 'Registers of John Gynewell, Bishop of Lincoln, for the years 1347–1350', *The Archaeological Journal*, LXVIII, 1911, pp. 300–360.

FISHER, J. L., 'The Black Death in Essex', *Essex Review*, LII, 1943, pp. 13–20.

KNIGHTON, HENRY, *Chronicon Henrici Knighton*, J. R. LUMBY, ed., vol. II. H.M.S.O., 1895.

LEVETT, A. E., 'The Black Death on the estates of the See of Winchester', p. 1–180, with a chapter on the manors of Witney, Brightwell, and Downton by A. BALLARD, p. 181–220, in VINOGRADOFF, P., ed., *Oxford Studies in Social and Legal History*, vol. 5, Clarendon Press, Oxford, 1916.

POSTAN, M. M., *Essays on Medieval Agriculture and General Problems of the Medieval Economy*, Cambridge University Press, 1973.

SEEBOHM, F., 'The Black Death, and its place in English History', *Fortnightly Review*, 2, 1865, pp. 149–160.

BAKER, ALAN R. H., 'Changes in the later Middle Ages', in DARBY, H. C., ed., *A New Historical Geography of England*, Cambridge University Press, 1973, pp. 186–247.

POSTAN, M. M. & TITOW, J., 'Heriots and prices on Winchester manors', *Economic History Review*, 2nd ser. II, 1958–9, pp. 392–411.

RUSSELL, J. C., 'Effects of Pestilence and Plague, 1315–1385', *Comparative Studies in Society and History*, 8, 1966, pp. 464–473.

HATCHER, JOHN, *Plague, Population and the English Economy 1348–1530*, Macmillan, London, 1977.

KOSMINSKY, E., 'The Evolution of Feudal Rent in England from the XIth to the XVth Centuries', *Past and Present*, 7, 1955, pp. 12–36.

GOTTFRIED, ROBERT S., *Epidemic Disease in Fifteenth Century England*, Leicester University Press, 1978.

ALLISON, K. J., 'The Lost Villages of Norfolk', *Norfolk Archaeology*, 31, 1955–7, pp. 116–162.

BERESFORD, M., '*The Lost Villages of England*', Lutterworth Press, London, 1954.

BERESFORD, M. W. & HURST, J. G., *Deserted Medieval Villages*, Lutterworth Press, London, 1971.

ALLISON, K. J., BERESFORD, M. W. & HURST, J. H., *The Deserted Villages of Oxfordshire*, Leicester University Press, 1965.

WILLIAMSON, R., 'The Plague in Cambridge', *Medical History*, 1, 1957, pp. 51–64.

SINGER, D. W., 'Some Plague Tractates (fourteenth and fifteenth centuries)', *Proceedings of the Royal Society of Medicine (Section of the History of Medicine)*, IX, 1916, pp. 159–212.

Chapter Five

HEINRICH, VON DIRK, 'Remarks on the Medieval Occurrence of the Norwegian rat (*Rattus norvegicus* Berkenhout, 1769) in Schleswig-Holstein', *Zoologischer Anzeiger, Jena*, 196, 1976, pp. 273–278.

BROWN, J. CLEVEDON & TWIGG, G. I., 'Studies on the Pelvis in British *Muridae* and *Cricetidae* (Rodentia)', *Journal of Zoology*, 158, 1969, pp. 81–132.

GESNER, *Book of Animals*, 1553.

THE BOOK OF KELLS, described by Sir Edward Sullivan, 3rd edn, 'The Studio' Limited, London, 1925.

FITTER, R. S. R., *The Ark in Our Midst*, Collins, London, 1959.

REFERENCES

GIRALDUS CAMBRENSIS, *Gemma Ecclesiastica*, vol. II of *Giraldus Cambrensis opera*, BREWER, J. S., ed., Longman, Green, Longman and Roberts, London, 1862.

GIRALDUS CAMBRENSIS, *The Itinerary through Wales and the Description of Wales*, J. M. Dent & Co., (Everyman), London, 1908.

PRYS-JONES, A. G., *Gerald of Wales. His 'Itinerary' through Wales and his 'Description' of the country and its people*, George G. Harrap & Co. Ltd., London, 1955.

BARRETT-HAMILTON, G. E. H., 'The Black or Ship Rat', in *A History of British Mammals*, Gurney & Jackson, London, 1913, pp. 578–599.

RUSSELL, J. C., 'That Earlier plague', *Demography*, 5, 1968, pp. 174–184.

HIRST, L. F., *'The Conquest of plague'*, Clarendon Press, Oxford, 1953.

BURNET, Sir MACFARLANE, *Natural History of Infectious Disease*, Cambridge University Press, 1962.

ZIEGLER, PHILIP, *The Black Death*, Pelican Books, England, 1970.

CHAPMAN, F. B., 'Exodus of Norway rats from flooded areas', *Journal of Mammalogy*, 19, 1938, pp. 376–377.

SHREWSBURY, J. F. D., *'A History of Bubonic Plague in the British Isles'*, Cambridge University Press, 1971.

TWIGG, GRAHAM, *The Brown Rat*, David and Charles, Newton Abbot, 1975.

RUSSELL, J. C., 'Effects of Pestilence and Plague, 1315–1385', *Comparative Studies in Society and History*, 8, 1966, pp. 464–473.

WING, L. W., 'Time Chart Measurements of Norwegian Lemming and Rodent Cycles', *Journal of Cycle Research*, 6, 1957, pp. 3–15.

WING, L. W., 'The 3.864-year Lemming Cycle and Latitudinal Passage in Temperature', *Journal of Cycle Research*, 10, 1961, pp. 57–70.

RACKHAM, J., *'Rattus rattus:* the introduction of the black rat into Britain', *Antiquity*, LIII, 1979, pp. 112–120.

NODDLE, BARBARA, 'The Animal Bones', in PLATT, COLIN & COLEMAN-SMITH, R. with others, *Excavations in medieval Southampton 1953–1969*, The excavation reports, Leicester University Press, vol. I pp. 332–339.

ARMITAGE, P. L., 'The mammalian remains from the Roman, medieval and early modern levels St. Magnus (New Fresh Wharf area III) London'. Unpublished level III archival report, Department of Urban Archaeology, Museum of London, 1979.

ARMITAGE, P. L., *The Mammalian Remains from the Tudor Site of Baynard's Castle, London: A Biometrical and Historical Analysis*, Ph.D. thesis, University of London, 1977.

ARMITAGE, P. L., WEST, B. & STEEDMAN, K., 'New Evidence of Black Rat in Roman London', *London Archaeologist* (in press), 1984.

O'CONNOR, T. P., 'Animal bones from Flaxengate, Lincoln, c. 870–1500', in *Archaeology of Lincoln*, vol. 18, pt. 1, Council for British Archaeology, London, 1982, pp. 40–41.

POLLITZER, R., *Plague. World Health Organization Monograph*, Series No. 22, Geneva, 1954.

DAVIS, D. E., 'The characteristics of rat populations', *Quarterly Review of Biology*, 28, 1953a, pp. 373–401.

MACARTHUR, W. P., 'The occurrence of the rat in early Europe', *Transactions of the Royal Society of Tropical Medicine and Hygiene*, 51, 1957, pp. 91–92.

SOUTHERN, H. N., *The Handbook of British Mammals*, Blackwell Scientific Publications, Oxford, 1964.

WHITE, T. H., ed., *The Book of Beasts. Being a translation from a Latin Bestiary of the twelfth century*, Jonathan Cape, London, 1954.

CAMPBELL, A. M., *The Black Death and Men of Learning*, New York, Columbia University Press, New York, 1931.

COULTON, G. G., *Life in the Middle Ages*, Cambridge University Press, 1930.

LANGLAND, W., *Piers Plowman. Text B*, DAVIS, J. F., ed., University Tutorial Press, London.

LANGLAND, W., *The Vision of William Concerning Piers the Plowman*, SKEAT, W. W., ed., Clarendon Press, Oxford, 1962.

CIPOLLA, C. M., *Cristofano and the Plague. A Study in the History of Public Health in the Age of Galileo*, Collins, London, 1973.

HANKIN, E. H., 'On the Epidemiology of Plague', *Journal of Hygiene*, 5, 1905, pp. 48–83.

DAVIS, D. H. S., 'Plague in South Africa: a study of the epizootic cycle in gerbils (*Tatera brantsi*) in the Northern Orange Free State', *Journal of Hygiene*, 51, 1953b, pp. 427–449.

PIRIE, J. H. H., 'Plague on the veld', *Publications of the South African Institute for Medical Research*, 3, 1927, pp. 138–162.

TWIGG, G. I., 'Infestations of the Brown Rat (*Rattus norvegicus*) in Drift Mines of the British Isles', *Journal of Hygiene*, 59, 1961, pp. 271–284.

BARNETT, S. A. & BATHARD, A. H., 'Population Dynamics of Sewer Rats', *Journal of Hygiene*, 51, 1953, pp. 483–491.

BENTLEY, E. W., BATHARD, A. H. & HAMMOND, L. E., 'Some Observations on a Rat Population in a Sewer', *Annals of Applied Biology*, 43, 1955, pp. 485–494.

BENTLEY, E. W., 'The Distribution and Status of *Rattus rattus* L. in the United Kingdom in 1951 and 1956', *Journal of Animal Ecology*, 28, 1959, pp. 299–308.

HERTER, K., 'Vorzugstemperaturen von Ratten und ihre ökologische Bedeutung', *Schädlingsbekämpfung*, 42, 1950, pp. 111–114.

REFERENCES

THOMSON, G. M., *The North-West Passage*, Secker & Warburg, London, 1975.

SCHILLER, E. L., 'Ecology and health of *Rattus* at Nome, Alaska', *Journal of Mammalogy*, 37, 1956, pp.181–188.

CORBET, G. B. & SOUTHERN, H. N., *The Handbook of British Mammals*, Blackwell Scientific Publications, Oxford, 1974.

MATHESON, C., 'A Survey of the Status of *Rattus rattus* and its Subspecies in the Seaports of Great Britain and Ireland', *Journal of Animal Ecology*, 8, 1939, pp.76–93.

PLAGUE RESEARCH COMMISSION, 'The Epidemiological Observations made by the Commission in Bombay City', *Journal of Hygiene*, 7, 1907, pp. 724–798.

AITKEN, E. H., 'Rats and the Plague', *Times of India*, 19 July 1899.

WATSON, J. S., 'Some Observations on the Reproduction of *Rattus rattus* L', *Proceedings of the Zoological Society of London*, 120, 1950, pp. 1–12.

FIGALA, J., 'The Reproduction and Population Structure of the Black rat, *Rattus rattus* (L.) in the Czechoslovak Habitats', *Acta Societatis Zoologicae Bohemoslovenicae*, XXVIII, 1964, pp. 48–67.

WATSON, J. S., 'The Rat Problem in Cyprus. A report of investigations made in carob-growing areas', *Colonial Research Publications*, No. 9, 1951, pp. 1–66. H.M.S.O.

LESLIE, P. H. & DAVIS, D. H. S., 'An Attempt to Determine the Absolute Number of Rats on a Given Area', *Journal of Animal Ecology*, 8, 1939, pp. 94–113.

Chapter Six

COULTON, G. G., *Medieval Panorama*, Cambridge University Press, 1949.

RUSSELL, J. C., *British Medieval Population*, The University of New Mexico Press, Albuquerque, 1948.

SHREWSBURY, J. F. D., *A History of Bubonic Plague in the British Isles*, Cambridge University Press, 1971.

ZIEGLER, PHILIP, *The Black Death*, Pelican Books, England, 1970.

ROGERS, J. E. THOROLD, *A History of Agriculture and Prices in England*, vol.1, *1259–1400*. Clarendon Press, Oxford, 1866.

BENNETT, H. S., *Life on the English Manor. A Study of Peasant Conditions, 1150–1400*, Cambridge University Press, 1938.

POSTAN, M. M., *The Medieval Economy and Society*, Pelican Books, England, 1975.

KOSMINSKY, E. A., *Studies in the Agrarian History of England in the Thirteenth Century*, HILTON, R. H., ed., translation by Ruth Kisch, Blackwell, Oxford, 1956.

HEIGHWAY, C. M., *The Erosion of History*, Council for British Archaeology, London, 1972.

LEVETT, A. E., 'The Black Death on the estates of the See of Winchester', p. 1–180, with a chapter on the manors of Witney, Brightwell, and Downton by A. BALLARD, p. 181–220, in VINOGRADOFF, P., ed., *Oxford Studies in Social and Legal History*, vol. 5, Clarendon Press, Oxford, 1916.

PLATT, COLIN, *Medieval England*, Routledge & Kegan Paul, London and Henley, 1978.

HOSKINS, W. G., *The Making of the English Landscape*, Book Club Associates, London, 1977.

RACKHAM, J., '*Rattus rattus*: the introduction of the black rat into Britain', *Antiquity*, LIII, 1979, pp. 112–120.

BLAIR, P. HUNTER, *Roman Britain and Early England 55 B.C. – A.D. 871*, Sphere Books Limited, London, 1970.

HILL, D. H., 'Continuity from Roman to Medieval: Britain', in *Origins of Towns*, part II of BARLEY, M. W., ed., *European towns. Their archaeology and early history*, Academic Press, London, 1977.

LOYN, H. R., *Anglo-Saxon England and the Norman conquest*, Longman, London, 1970.

MORRIS, J., *The Age of Arthur. A history of the British Isles from 350 to 650*, Weidenfeld and Nicholson, London, 1973.

ALCOCK, LESLIE, *Arthur's Britain*, Penguin Books Ltd., Harmondsworth, 1971.

TANSLEY, A. G., *Britain's Green Mantle: Past, Present and Future*, George Allen and Unwin Ltd, London, 1968.

TITOW, J. Z., 'Some Evidence of the Thirteenth Century Population Increase', *Economic History Review*, 2nd Series, XIV, 1961–2, pp. 218–224.

HARVEY, BARBARA F., 'The Population Trend in England between 1300 and 1348', *Transactions of the Royal Historical Society*, 16, 1966, pp. 23–42.

RUSSELL, J. C., 'The Preplague Population of England', *Journal of British Studies*, V. 1966, pp. 1–21.

HALLAM, H. E., 'Population Density in Medieval Fenland', *Economic History Review*, 2nd Series, XIV, 1961–2, pp. 71–81.

HALLAM, H. H., 'Some Thirteenth-Century Censuses', *Economic History Review*, 2nd Series, X, 1957–8, pp. 340–361.

BENTLEY, E. W., 'The Distribution and Status of *Rattus rattus* L. in the United Kingdom in 1951 and 1956'. *Journal of Animal Ecology*, 28, 1959, pp. 299–308.

BIDDLE, M., 'The Evolution of Towns: Planned Towns before 1066', in BARLEY, M. W., ed., *The Plans and Topography of Medieval Towns in England and Wales*, The Council for British Archaeology, 1976, pp. 19–32.

BERESFORD, MAURICE, *New towns of the Middle Ages. Town plantation in England, Wales and Gascony*, Lutterworth Press, London, 1967.

BUTLER, L., 'The Evolution of Towns: Planted Towns after 1066', in BARLEY, M. W., ed., *The Plans and Topography of Medieval Towns in England and Wales*, The Council for British Archaeology, 1976, pp. 32–48.

PLATT, C., 'The Evolution of Towns: Natural Growth', in BARLEY, M. W., ed., *The Plans and Topography of Medieval Towns in England and Wales*, The Council for British Archaeology, 1976, pp. 48–56.

TOUT, T. F., 'Mediaeval Town Planning', *The Bulletin of the John Rylands Library*, vol. 4, No. 1, April–August, 1917.

SLATER, GILBERT, 'The Inclosure of Common Fields Considered Geographically', *Geographical Journal*, XXIX, 1907, pp. 35–55.

POSTAN, M. M., *The Medieval Economy and Society*, Penguin Books Ltd., Harmondsworth, 1975.

NEILSON, NELLIE, 'Medieval Agrarian Society in its Prime: England', in CLAPHAM, J. H., & POWER, E., eds, *The Cambridge Economic History of Europe*, vol. 1, Cambridge University Press, 1941, pp. 438–466.

CLIFTON-TAYLOR, ALEC, *The Pattern of English Building*, Faber and Faber Limited, London, 1972.

MUIR, RICHARD, *The English Village*, Thames and Hudson Limited, London, 1980.

BERESFORD, M. W. & HURST, J. C., 'Wharram Percy: a case study in microtopography', in SAWYER, P. H., ed., *English Medieval Settlement*, Edward Arnold, London, 1979, pp. 52–85.

ROWLEY, TREVOR, *Villages in the Landscape*, J. M. Dent & Sons Ltd., London, 1978.

COULTON, G. G., *The Medieval Village*, Cambridge University Press, 1925.

GASQUET, F. A., *The Black Death of 1348 and 1349*, George Bell and Sons, London, 1908.

EDWARDS, TUDOR, *The Ancient Stones of England*, Robert Hale, London, 1972.

PEATE, IORWERTH C., *The Welsh House. A study in folk culture*, Hugh Evans & Sons, Ltd, Liverpool, 1944.

HARVEY, P. D. A., *A Medieval Oxfordshire Village. Cuxham, 1240 to 1400*, Oxford University Press, 1965.

PLATT, COLIN, *Medieval Southampton. The port and trading community*, A.D. 1000–1600, Routledge & Kegan Paul, London, 1973.

WILSON, DAVID M. & HURST, D. GILLIAN, 'Medieval Britain in 1962 and 1963. Northamptonshire: Northampton Castle', *Medieval Archaeology*, 8, 1964, pp. 257–258.

WEBSTER, LESLIE E. & CHERRY, JOHN, 'Medieval Britain in 1974. Kent: Hythe', *Medieval Archaeology*, 19, 1975, p. 245.

WEBSTER, LESLIE E. & CHERRY, JOHN, 'Medieval Britain in 1973. Northamptonshire: Northampton', *Medieval Archaeology*, 18, 1974, p. 202.

CARTER, A., ROBERTS, J. P. & SUTERMEISTER, HELENA, 'Excavations in Norwich – 1973. The Norwich Survey – Third Interim Report', *Norwich Archaeology*, 36, 1977, pp. 39–71.

PLAGUE RESEARCH COMMISSION, 'Observations on plague in Belgaum, 1908–1909', *Journal of Hygiene*, 10, 1910, pp. 446–482.

DAVIS, D. E., 'The Rat Population of New York, 1949', *American Journal of Hygiene*, 52, 1950, pp. 147–152.

DAVIS, D. E., & FALES, W. T., 'The Rat Population of Baltimore, 1949', *American Journal of Hygiene*, 52, 1950, pp. 142–146.

PETRIE, G. F. & TODD, R. E., 'A Report on Plague Investigations in Egypt', *Reports and Notes of the Public Health Laboratories, Cairo*, 5, 1923, pp. 1–114.

SABINE, E. L., 'Latrines and Cesspools of Mediaeval London', *Speculum*, IX, 1934, pp. 303–321.

SABINE, E. L., 'Butchering in Mediaeval London', *Speculum*, VIII, 1933, pp. 335–352.

WILLIAMSON, R., 'The Plague in Cambridge', *Medical History*, 1, 1957, pp. 51–64.

SABINE, E. L., 'City cleaning in Mediaeval London', *Speculum*, XII, 1937, pp. 19–43.

HENSCHEN, F., *The History of Diseases*, Longmans, Green & Co. Ltd, London, 1966.

PHILIP, W. M. & HIRST, L. F., 'A Report on the Outbreak of the Plague in Colombo, 1914–1916', *Journal of Hygiene*, 15, 1917, pp. 527–564.

Chapter Seven

MEAD-BRIGGS, A. R. & RUDGE, A. J. B., 'Breeding of the Rabbit Flea, *Spilopsyllus cuniculi* (Dale); requirement of a 'factor' from a pregnant rabbit for ovarian maturation', *Nature*, 187, 1960, pp. 1136–1137.

ROTHSCHILD, M. & FORD, B., 'Reproductive Hormones of the Host Controlling the Sexual Cycle of the Rabbit Flea (*Spilopsyllus cuniculi* Dale)', *Proceedings of the International Congress of Entomology*, 12, London (1964), 1966, pp. 801–802.

BACOT, A. W., 'A Study fo the Bionomics of the Common Rat Fleas and Other Species Associated with Human Habitations, with special reference to the influence of temperature and humidity at various periods of the life history of the insect', *Journal of Hygiene*, 13, 1914, pp. 447–654.

PETRIE, G. F. & TODD, R. E., 'A Report on plague investigations in Egypt', *Reports and Notes of the Public Health Laboratories, Cairo*, 5, 1923, pp. 1–114.

REFERENCES

HIRST, L. F., 'Rat-flea Surveys and their Use as a Guide to Plague Preventive Measures', *Transactions of the Royal Society of Tropical Medicine and Hygiene*, 21, 1927–8, pp. 87–104.

PLAGUE RESEARCH COMMISSION, 'On the Seasonal Prevalence of Plague in India', *Journal of Hygiene*, 8, 1908, pp. 266–301.

PLAGUE RESEARCH COMMISSION, 'Observations on Plague in Poona', *Journal of Hygiene*, 10, 1910, pp. 483–535.

PLAGUE RESEARCH COMMISSION, 'Observations on Plague in Belgaum', *Journal of Hygiene*, 10, 1910a, pp. 446–482.

PLAGUE RESEARCH COMMISSION, 'Statistical Investigation of Plague in the Punjab. Third Report: on some of the factors which influence the prevalence of plague', *Journal of Hygiene*, 11, 1911, pp. 62–156.

GLOSTER, T. H. & WHITE, F. N., 'Epidemiological Observations in the United Provinces of Agra and Oudh, 1911–1912', *Journal of Hygiene*, 15, 1917, pp. 793–880.

BROOKS, R. ST.-J. 'The Influence of Saturation Deficiency and of Temperature on the Course of Epidemic Plague', *Journal of Hygiene*, 15, 1917, pp. 881–899.

SHREWSBURY, J. F. D., *A History of bubonic plague in the British Isles*, Cambridge University Press, 1971.

POLLITZER, R., *Plague. World Health Organization Monograph*, Series No. 22, Geneva, 1954.

LAMB, H. H., *The Changing Climate*, Methuen, London, 1966.

UTTERSTRÖM, G., 'Climatic Fluctuations and Population Problems in Early Modern History', *Scandinavian Economic History Review*, III, 1955, pp. 3–47.

LAMB, H. H., *Climate present, past and future*, Methuen, London, 1977.

MANLEY, G., 'The climate of the British Isles', in, WALLEN, C. C., ed., *Climates of Northern and Western Europe*, vol. 5 of *World Survey of Climatology*, Amsterdam, 1970, pp. 81–133.

ARLÉRY, R., 'The climate of France, Belgium, the Netherlands and Luxembourg', in WALLEN, C. C., ed., *Climates of Northern and Western Europe*, vol. 5 of *World Survey of Climatology*, Elsevier Publishing Company, Amsterdam, 1970, pp. 135–193.

SHIPLEY, A. E., 'Rat fleas', *Journal of Economic Biology*, VI, 1911, pp. 12–20.

COULTON, G. G., *Mediaeval Panorama*, Cambridge University Press, 1949.

ROUBAUD, E., 'Foyer de développement de *Xenopsylla cheopis* à Paris. Observations sur la Biologie de cette puce', *Bulletin de la Société de Pathologie Exotique*, 21, 1928, pp. 227–230.

GIRARD, G., 'Présence de *Xenopsylla cheopis* sur les rats noirs capturés a Paris', *Bulletin de la Société de Pathologie Exotique*, 39, 1946, pp. 365–367.

JORDAN, K. & ROTHSCHILD, The Hon. N. C., 'Revision of the non-combed eyed *Siphonaptera*', *Parasitology*, 1, 1908, pp. 1–100.

JORDAN, K., 'On Some *Siphonaptera* from Tropical Africa and Iraq', *Novitates Zoologicae*, 41, 1938–9, pp. 112–118.

TOUMANOFF, C. & HERIVAUX, A. 'La nature du sol et le stationnement des puces (*X. cheopis* et *X. astia*). Essai d'interprétation', *Bulletin de la Société de Pathologie Exotique*, 41, 1948, pp. 293–300.

HIRST, L. F., 'A Rat-flea Survey of Ceylon', *Ceylon Journal of Science (Section D)*, 3, 1933–5, pp. 48–113.

KING, H. H. & PANDIT, C. G., 'A summary of the rat-flea survey of the Madras Presidency with a discussion on the association of flea species with climate and with plague', *Indian Journal of Medical Research*, 19, 1931, pp. 357–392.

MACARTHUR, W. P., 'Old-time plague in Britain', *Transactions of the Royal Society of Tropical Medicine and Hygiene*, 19, 1926, pp. 355–372.

ESKEY, C. R. & HAAS, V. H., 'Plague in the Western Part of the United States', *United States Public Health Service, Public Health Bulletin* No. 254, 1940, pp. 1–83.

ESKEY, C. R., 'Recent Developments in our Knowledge of Plague Transmission', *Public Health Reports, Washington*, 53, 1938a, pp. 49–58.

ESKEY, C. R., 'Fleas as Vectors of Plague', *American Journal of Public Health*, 28, 1938b, pp. 1305–1310.

DOUGLAS, J. R. & WHEELER, C. M., 'Sylvatic Plague Studies. II. The fate of *Pasteurella pestis* in the flea', *Journal of Infectious Diseases*, 72, 1943, pp. 18–30.

PLAGUE RESEARCH COMMISSION, 'The Mechanism by Means of Which the Flea Clears Itself of Plague Bacilli', *Journal of Hygiene*, 8, 1908a, pp. 260–265.

LEDINGHAM, J. C. G., 'The Influence of Temperature on Phagocytosis', *Proceedings of the Royal Society, B*, LXXX, 1908, pp. 188–195.

HIRST, L. F., *The protection of the interior of Ceylon from plague with special reference to the fumigation of plague-suspect imports*, Colombo, 1931.

JORDAN, K., 'Fleas', in SMART, J., *A Handbook for the Identification of Insects of Medical Importance*, by order of the Trustees of the British Museum, London, 1948, pp. 211–245.

Chapter Eight

GILL, C. A., *The Genesis of Epidemics and the natural history of disease*, Baillière, Tindall and Cox, London, 1928.

PLAGUE RESEARCH COMMISSION, 'Observations made in Four Villages in the Neighbourhood of Bombay', *Journal of Hygiene*, 7, 1907, pp. 799–873.

PETRIE, G. F. & TODD, R. E., 'A Report on Plague Investigations in Egypt', *Reports and Notes of the Public Health Laboratories, Cairo*, 5, 1923, pp. 1–114.

DAVIS, D. E., EMLEN, J. T. & STOKES, A. W., 'Studies on Home Range in the Brown Rat', *Journal of Mammalogy*, 29, 1948, pp. 207–225.

REFERENCES

DAVIS, D. E., 'The Characteristics of Rat Populations', *Quarterly Review of Biology*, 28, 1953, pp. 373–401.

WATSON, J. S., 'The Rat Problem in Cyprus. A report of investigations made in carob-growing areas', *Colonial Research Publications*, No. 9, 1951, pp. 1–66, H.M.S.O.

TOMICH, P. Q., 'Movement Patterns of Field Rodents in Hawaii', *Pacific Science*, XXIV, 1970, pp. 195–234.

AITKEN, E. H., 'Rats and the Plague', *Times of India*, 19 July 1899.

SHREWSBURY, J. F. D., *A History of Bubonic Plague in the British Isles*. Cambridge University Press, 1971.

SIMPSON, W. J., *A Treatise on Plague Dealing with the Historical, Epidemiological, Clinical, Therapeutic and Preventive Aspects of the Disease*, Cambridge University Press, 1905.

MITCHELL, J. A., 'Plague in South Africa: historical summary', *Publications of the South African Institute for Medical Research*, 3, 1927, pp. 89–104.

LANGER, W. L., 'The Black Death', *Scientific American*, 210, 1964, pp. 114–121.

MITCHELL, J. A., 'Plague in South Africa: perpetuation and spread of infection by wild rodents', *Journal of Hygiene*, 20, 1921, pp. 377–382.

ESKEY, C. R., 'Epidemiological Study of Plague in the Hawaiian Islands', *United States Public Health Service, Public Health Bulletin*, No. 213, 1934, pp. 1–70.

GROSS, B. & BONNET, D. D., 'Plague in the Territory of Hawaii. I. Present status of plague infection, Island of Hawaii', *Public Health Report*, 66, 1951, pp. 209–214.

ESKEY, C. R. & HAAS, V. H., 'Plague in the Western Part of the United States', *United States Public Health Service, Public Health Bulletin*, No. 254, 1940, pp. 1–83.

ELL, STEPHEN R., 'Some Evidence for Interhuman Transmission of Medieval Plague', *Reviews of Infectious Diseases*, 1, 1979, pp. 563–566.

BALTAZARD, M., BAHMANYAR, M., MOSTACHFI, P., EFTEKHARI, M. & MOFIDI, Ch., 'Recherches sur la peste en Iran', *Bulletin of the World Health Organization*, 23, 1960, pp. 141–155.

BALTAZARD, M., 'Déclin et Destin d'une Maladie infectieuse: la Peste', *Bulletin of the World Health Organization*, 23, 1960, pp. 247–262.

WU, LIEN-TEH, CHUN, J. W. H., POLLITZER, R. & WU, C. Y., *Plague: A manual for medical and public health workers*, National Quarantine Service, Shanghai Station, China, 1936.
New Scientist, 94, 1982, p. 492.

MARTIN, C. J., 'The Spread of Plague', *British Medical Journal*, 11 Nov. 1911, pp. 1–35.

BURNET, Sir MACFARLANE, *Natural history of Infectious Disease*, Cambridge University Press, 1962.

Chapter Nine

LOW, R. BRUCE, *Reports and Papers on Bubonic Plague. An account of the progress and diffusion of plague throughout the world, 1898–1901, and of the measures employed in different countries for repression of this disease*, H.M.S.O., 1902.

HIRST, L. F., *The Conquest of Plague*, Clarendon Press, Oxford, 1953.

H.M.S.O., 'Reports and Papers on Suspected Cases of Human Plague in East Suffolk and on an Epizootic of Plague in Rodents', in *Reports to the Local Government Board on Public Health and Medical Subjects* (New Series, No. 52), H.M.S.O., 1911, pp. 1–87.

PLAGUE RESEARCH COMMISSION, 'Observations in the Punjab Villages of Dhand and Kasel', *Journal of Hygiene*, 7, 1907, pp. 895–994.

TIRABOSCHI, C., 'Les Rats, les Souris et leurs parasites cutanés dans leurs rapports avec la propagation de la peste bubonique', *Archives de Parasitologie*, VIII, 1903–4, pp. 161–349.

TIRABOSCHI, C., 'État actuel de la question du véhicule de la peste', *Archives de Parasitologie*, XI, 1906–7, p. 545–620.

ROTHSCHILD, the Hon. N. CHARLES, 'Note on the species of fleas found upon rats, *Mus rattus* and *Mus decumanus*, in different parts of the world, and on some variations in the proportion of each species in different localities', *Journal of Hygiene*, 6, 1906, pp. 483–485.

VERJBITSKI, D. T., 'The Part played by Insects in the Epidemiology of Plague', *Journal of Hygiene*, 8, 1908, pp. 162–208.

ROTHSCHILD, The Hon. N. CHARLES, 'A Synopsis of the Fleas Found on *Mus norwegicus decumanus*, *Mus rattus Alexandrinus* and *Mus musculus*', *Bulletin of Entomological Research*, 1, 1910, pp. 89–98.

BALFOUR, A., 'Observations on Wild Rats in England, with an account of their ecto- and endoparasites', *Parasitology*, 14, 1922, pp. 282–298.

SHREWSBURY, J. F. D., *A History of Bubonic Plague in the British Isles*, Cambridge University Press, 1971.

PETRIE, G. F. & TODD, R. E., 'A Report on Plague Investigations in Egypt', *Reports and Notes of the Public Health Laboratories, Cairo*, 5, 1923, pp. 1–114.

SEAL, S. C., 'Epidemiological Studies of Plague in India. 1. The present position', *Bulletin of the World Health Organization*, 23, 1969, pp. 283–292.

WU, LIEN-TEH, *A Treatise on Pneumonic Plague*, The League of Nations, Geneva, 1926.

WU, LIEN-TEH, 'Plague in the Orient with special reference to the Manchurian outbreaks', *Journal of Hygiene*, 26, 1922, pp. 62–76.

BANNERMAN, W. B., 'The Spread of Plague in India', *Journal of Hygiene*, 6, 1906, pp. 179–211.

BLOUNT, R. E., 'Plague', in *Tropical Medicine*, HUNTER, G. W.,

REFERENCES

SWARTZWELDER, J. C. & CLYDE, D. F., eds, W. B. Saunders Co., Philadelphia, 1976, pp. 224–233.

MORRIS, CHRISTOPHER, 'The Plague in Britain', *The Historical Journal*, XIV, 1971, pp. 205–215.

SHREWSBURY, J. F. D., *The Plague of the Philistines and other medical essays*, Victor Gollancz Ltd, London, 1964.

WU, LIEN-TEH, CHUN, J. W. H., POLLITZER, R. & WU, C. Y., *Plague: A manual for medical and public health workers*, National Quarantine Service, Shanghai Station, China, 1936.

LAFONT, A., 'Une épidémie de peste humaine à Dakar (avril 1914 – février 1915)', *Bulletin de la Société de Pathologie Exotique*, 8, 1915, pp. 660–680.

TWIGG, G. I., 'A Review of the Occurrence in British Mammals of the Major Organisms of Zoonotic Importance', *Mammal Review*, 10, 1980, pp. 139–149.

Chapter Ten

PLAGUE RESEARCH COMMISSION, 'Digest of Recent Observations on the Epidemiology of Plague', *Journal of Hygiene*, 7, 1907, pp. 694–723.

INDIAN PLAGUE COMMISSION, *Indian Plague Commission, 1898–99*, H.M.S.O., 1901, vol. 5, p. 132.

WU, LIEN-TEH, CHUN, J. W. H., POLLITZER, R. & WU, C. Y., *Plague: A manual for medical and public health workers*, National Quarantine Service, Shanghai Station, China, 1936.

BROWNLEE, J., 'Certain Aspects of the Theory of Epidemiology in Special Relation to Plague', *Proceedings of the Royal Society of Medicine* (Section of Epidemiology and State Medicine), XI, 1918, pp. 85–132.

PLAGUE RESEARCH COMMISSION, 'The Epidemiological Observations made by the Commission in Bombay City', *Journal of Hygiene*, 7, 1907a, pp. 724–798.

ZIEGLER, PHILIP, *The Black Death*, Pelican Books, England, 1970.
SHREWSBURY, J. F. D., *A History of Bubonic Plague in the British Isles*, Cambridge University Press, 1971.

REES, W, 'The Black Death in England and Wales, as Exhibited in Manorial Documents', *Proceedings of the Royal Society of Medicine* (Section of the History of Medicine), XVI, 1923, pp. 27–45.

LUNN, J., 'The Black Death in the Bishop's Registers', unpublished typescript copy of a thesis awarded the Ph.D. degree of Cambridge University, 1937.

CREIGHTON, C., *A History of Epidemics in Britain*, 1894, 2nd edn., with additional material by D. E. C. EVERSLEY, E. A. UNDERWOOD and L. OVENALL, Frank Cass & Co. Ltd, London, 1965.

GASQUET, F. A., *The Black Death of 1348 and 1349*, George Bell and Sons, London, 1908.

FLETCHER, J. M. J., 'The Black Death in Dorset, (1348–1349)', *Dorset Natural History and Antiquarian Field Club*, Vol. XLIII, 1922, pp. 1–14.

RUSSELL, J. C., *British Medieval Population*, The University of New Mexico Press, Albuquerque, 1948.

THOMPSON, A. HAMILTON, 'Registers of John Gynewell, Bishop of Lincoln, for the years 1347–1350', *The Archaeological Journal*, LXVIII, 1911, pp. 300–360.

THOMPSON, A. HAMILTON, 'The Pestilences of the Fourteenth Century in the Diocese of York', *The Archaeological Journal*, LXXI, 1914, pp. 97–154.

LEVETT, A. E., *The Black Death on the St. Albans Manors. Studies in Manorial History*, Clarendon Press, Oxford, 1938.

TITOW, J., 'Evidence of Weather in the Account Rolls of the Bishop of Winchester 1209–1350', *Economic History Review*, 2nd Series, XII, 1959–60, pp. 360–407.

GREENWOOD, M., 'Part II. Statistical Analyses of Data Respecting Epidemics of Bubonic Plague in Three Districts of the Punjab', *Journal of Hygiene*, 10, 1910, pp. 416–443.

PLAGUE RESEARCH COMMISSION, 'Observations in the Punjab Villages of Dhand and Kasel', *Journal of Hygiene*, 7, 1907b, pp. 895–985.

HIRST, L. F., *The Conquest of plague*, Clarendon Press, Oxford, 1953.

ENNEN, EDITH, *The Medieval Town*, vol. 15 of *Europe in the Middle Ages: Selected Studies*, VAUGHAN, R. ed., North Holland Publishing Company, Amsterdam, 1979.

BATH B. H. SLICHER VAN, *The Agrarian History of Western Europe* A.D. *500–1850*, Edward Arnold, London, 1963.

POSTAN, M. M. & TITOW, J., 'Heriots and Prices on Winchester Manors', *Economic History Review*, 2nd Series, II 1958–9, pp. 392–411.

WOOD, W., *The History and Antiquities of Eyam: with a minute account of the Great Plague which desolated that village in the year 1666*, 4th edn, Richard Keene, Derby, 1865.

MEAD, RICHARD, *A Discourse on the Plague*, 9th edn, London, 1744.
The diary of Samuel Pepys, vol. 2, ed. from Mynors Bright, J. M. Dent & Sons Ltd, London, 1953.

BRADLEY, LESLIE, 'The Most Famous of all English Plagues', in *The Plague Reconsidered*, A Local Population Studies Supplement, pp. 63–94.

PETRIE, G. F. & TODD, R. E., 'A Report on Plague Investigations in Egypt', *Reports and Notes of the Public Health Laboratories, Cairo*, 5, 1923, pp. 1–114.

BRETT-JAMES, N. G., *The Growth of Stuart London*, George Allen & Unwin Ltd, London, 1935.

SEAL, S. C., 'Epidemiological Studies of Plague in India. 1. The present position', *Bulletin of the World Health Organization*, 23, 1969, pp. 283–292.

LOW, R. BRUCE, 'An account of the progress and diffusion of plague throughout the world, 1898–1901, and of the measures employed in different countries for repression of this disease', *Reports and papers on bubonic plague*, H.M.S.O., 1902.

GILL, C. A., *The Genesis of Epidemics and the Natural History of Disease*, Baillière, Tindall and Cox, London, 1928.

ROBERTUS DE AVESBURY, *De Gestis Mirabilibus Regis Edwardi Tertii*, THOMPSON, EDWARD MAUNDE, ed., H.M.S.O. 1889.

Chapter Eleven

BONSER, W., 'Epidemics during the Anglo-Saxon Period', *Journal of the British Archaeological Association*, 3rd Series, 9, 1944, pp. 48–71.

MACARTHUR, Sir WILLIAM, 'Famine Fevers in England and Ireland', appendix, p. 66–71 to BONSER, W., 'Epidemics during the Anglo-Saxon Period', *Journal of the British Archaeological Association*, 3rd Ser., 9, 1944, pp. 48–71.

CREIGHTON, C., *A History of Epidemics in Britain*, 1894 2nd edn., with additional material by D. E. C. EVERSLEY, E. A. UNDERWOOD and L. OVENALL, Frank Cass & Co. Ltd, London, 1965.

LUCAS, H. S., 'The Great European Famine of 1315, 1316 and 1317', *Speculum*, 5, 1930, pp. 343–377.

MACARTHUR, W. 'The Medical Identification of Some Pestilences of the Past', *Transactions of the Royal Society of Tropical Medicine and Hygiene*, 53, 1959, pp. 423–439.

BOUCHER, C. E., 'The Black Death in Bristol', *Transactions of the Bristol and Gloucestershire Archaeological Society*, Vol. LX, 1938, pp. 31–46.

HOWE, C. MELVYN, *Man, Environment and Disease in Britain*, David & Charles, Newton Abbot, 1972.

GASQUET, F. A., *The Black Death of 1348 and 1349*, George Bell and Sons, London, 1908.

PONTANUS, J. J., *Rerum Danicarum Historia*, 1631 (p. 476 in Gasquet, 1908).

ANGLADA, A., *Étude sur les Maladies Éteintes*, Paris, 1869.

HECKER, J. F. C. *The Epidemics of the Middle Ages*, translated by B. G. Babington, 3rd edn, Trübner & Co., London, 1859.

BARTSOCAS, CHRISTOS S., 'Two Fourteenth Century Greek Descriptions of the "Black Death" ', *Journal of the History of Medicine*, XXI, 1966, pp. 394–400.

MICHAEL PLATIENSIS, *Bibliotheca Scriptorum Qui Res in Sicilia Gestas Retulere*, vol. 1, p. 562.

NOHL, JOHANNES, *The Black Death: A chronicle of the plague*. George Allen & Unwin Ltd, London, 1926.

THOMPSON, EDWARD MAUNDE, ed., *Chronicon Galfridi le Baker de Swynebroke*, Clarendon Press, Oxford, 1889.

SHREWSBURY, J. F. D., *A History of Bubonic Plague in the British Isles*, Cambridge University Press, 1971.

MACARTHUR, W. P., 'Old-time Plague in Britain', *Transactions of the Royal Society of Tropical Medicine and Hygiene*, 19, 1926, pp. 355–372.

CHRISTIE, A. B. *Infectious Diseases: Epidemiology and Clinical Practice*, 3rd edn, Churchill Livingstone, Edinburgh, London & New York, 1980.

IMPERATO, P. J. *The Treatment and Control of Infectious Diseases in Man*, Charles C. Thomas, Springfield, Illinois, 1974.

CRUICKSHANK, R., *Medical Microbiology. A guide to the laboratory diagnosis and control of infection*, English Language Book Society and E. & S. Livingstone Ltd, 1965.

MAIR, N. S., 'Pseudotuberculosis in Free-living Wild Animals', *Symposia of the Zoological Society of London*, No. 24, 1968, pp. 107–117.

D'IRSAY, S., 'Defense Reactions during the Black Death, 1348–1349', *Annals of Medical History*, 9, 1927, pp. 169–179.

LECLAINCHE, E., *Histoire de la Médecine Vétérinaire*, Office du Livre, Toulouse, 1936.

REES, W. 'The Black Death in England and Wales, as Exhibited in Manorial Documents', *Proceedings of the Royal Society of Medicine* (Section of the History of Medicine), XVI, 1923, pp. 27–45.

KNIGHTON, HENRY, *Chronicon Henrici Knighton*, LUMBY, J. R., ED., H.M.S.O., 1889–95.

THOMAS WALSINGHAM, *Historia Anglicana*, Rolls Ser., RILEY, H. T., ed., Longman, Green, Longman, Roberts and Green, London, 1863 vol. I, p. 309.

SKEYNE, GILBERT, *Ane Breve Descriptioun of the Pest (etc.)* Edinburgh, 1568.

SIMPSON, W. J., *A Treatise on Plague dealing with the Historical, Epidemiological, Clinical, Therapeutic and Preventive Aspects of the Disease*, Cambridge University Press, 1905.

LIDDELL, H. G. & SCOTT, R., *A Greek-English Lexicon*, Clarendon Press, Oxford, 1968.

The Anglo-Saxon Chronicle, Translation by Garmonsway, G. N., J. M. Dent & Sons Ltd, London, 1955.

MEAD, RICHARD, *A Practical Treatise of the Plague and all Pestilential Infections that have happen'd in this Island for the last Century*, London, 1720.

HARVEY, P. D. A., *A Medieval Oxfordshire Village. Cuxham, 1240 to 1400*, Oxford University Press, 1965.

SABINE, E. L., 'Butchering in Mediaeval London', *Speculum*, VIII, 1933, pp. 335–352.

REFERENCES

HARROD, HENRY, 'Some Details of a Murrain of the Fourteenth Century; from the Court Rolls of a Norfolk Manor', *Archaeologia*, XLI, 1867, pp. 1--14.

ADAMNAN (Saint), *The Life of Saint Columba (Columb-Kille)* A.D. *521–597*, translation by Wentworth Huyshe (1906), George Routledge & Sons, Limited, London.

GREGORY OF TOURS, *The History of the Franks*, (2 vols., translation by O. M. Dalton, Clarendon Press, Oxford, 1927, I, 421–2; II, 119, 141, 395, 516, 600.

COULTON, G. G., *Life in the Middle Ages*, Cambridge University Press, 1930, vol. IV, p. 209.

PROTHERO, R. E. (1st Baron Ernle), *English Farming Past and Present*, Longmans, Green and Co., London, 1919.

POWER, EILEEN, *The Wool Trade in English Medieval History*, Oxford University Press, 1941.

LLOYD, T. H., *The English Wool Trade in the Middle Ages*, Cambridge University Press, 1977.

PELHAM, R. A. 'Fourteenth Century England', in DARBY, H. C., ed., *An historical geography of England before* A.D. *1800*, Cambridge University Press, 1951, pp. 230–265.

ROGERS, J. E. THOROLD, *A History of Agriculture and Prices in England*, vol. I, *1259–1400*. Clarendon Press, Oxford, 1866.

DONKIN, R. A. 'Cattle on the Estates of Cistercian Monasteries in England and Wales', *Economic History Review*, 2nd Series, XV, 1962–3, pp. 31–53.

POSTAN, M. M., Village livestock in the Thirteenth Century, *Economic History Review*, 2nd Series, XV, 1962–3, pp. 219–249.

KERSHAW, IAN, 'The Great Famine and Agrarian Crisis in England 1315–1322', *Past and Present*, No. 59, 1973, pp. 3–50.

FINBERG, H. P. R., *Tavistock Abbey. A study in the social and economic history of Devon*, Cambridge University Press, 1951.

ENNEN, EDITH, *The Medieval Town*, vol. 15 of *Europe in the Middle Ages: Selected Studies*, VAUGHAN, R., ed., North Holland Publishing Company, Amsterdam, 1979.

VEALE, ELSPETH, M., *The English Fur Trade in the Later Middle Ages*, Clarendon Press, Oxford, 1966.

WOOD, W., *The History and Antiquities of Eyam: with a minute account of the Great Plague which desolated that village in the year 1666*, 4th edn, Richard Keene, Derby, 1865.

HURST, G. W., 'Foot-and-mouth Disease. The possibility of continental sources of the virus in England in epidemics of October 1967 and several other years', *Veterinary Record*, 82, 1968, pp. 610–614.

SELLERS, R. F. & PARKER, J., 'Airborne excretion of foot-and-mouth disease virus', *Journal of Hygiene*, 67, 1969, pp. 671–77.

HENDERSON, R. J. 'The outbreak of foot-and-mouth disease in Worcestershire. An epidemiological study: with special reference to spread of the disease by wind-carriage of the virus', *Journal of Hygiene*, 67, 1969, pp. 21–33.

TINLINE, R., 'Lee wave hypothesis for the initial pattern of spread during the 1967–68 foot and mouth epizootic', *Nature*, 227, 1970, pp. 860–62.

ZIEGLER, PHILIP, *The Black Death*, Pelican Books, England, 1970.

Bibliography

Major works on plague and disease

BIRABEN, JEAN-NOËL, *Les hommes et la peste en France et dans les pays européens et mediterranéens*, tome 1 of *La peste dans l'histoire*, Mouton & Co. and Ecole des Hautes Etudes en Sciences Sociales, 1975.

BOWSKY, W. M., ed., *The Black Death; A Turning Point in History?*, Robert E. Krieger Publishing Company, New York, 1978.

CREIGHTON, C., *A History of Epidemics in Britain*, 1894, 2nd edn, with additional material by D. E. C. EVERSLEY, E. A. UNDERWOOD and L. OVENALL, Frank Cass & Co. Ltd, London 1965.

GASQUET, F. A., *The Black Death of 1348 and 1349*, George Bell and Sons, London, 1908.

GILL, C. A., *The Genesis of Epidemics and the Natural History of Disease*, Baillière, Tindall & Cox, London, 1928.

GOTTFRIED, ROBERT S., *Epidemic disease in Fifteenth Century England*, Leicester University Press, 1978.

GOTTFRIED, ROBERT S., *The Black Death: Natural and Human Disaster in Medieval Europe*, Robert Hall/Macmillan, London, 1983.

HATCHER, JOHN, *Plague, Population and the English Economy 1348–1530*, Macmillan, London, 1977.

HECKER, J. F. C., *The Epidemics of the Middle Ages*, translated by B. G. Babington, 3rd edn., Trübner & Co., London, 1859.

HENSCHEN, F., *The History of Diseases*, Longmans, Green & Co. Ltd., London, 1966.

HIRST, L. F., *The Conquest of Plague*, Clarendon Press, Oxford, 1953.

McNEILL, W. H., *Plagues and Peoples*, Blackwell, Oxford, 1977.

NOHL, JOHANNES, *The Black Death: A chronicle of the plague*, George Allen & Unwin Ltd., London 1926.

POLLITZER, R., *Plague. World Health Organization Monograph*, Series No. 22, Geneva, 1954.

Reports on Plague Investigations in India, 1906–17. *Journal of Hygiene.*

SHREWSBURY, J. F. D., *A History of Bubonic Plague in the British Isles*, Cambridge University Press, 1971.

SIMPSON, W. J., *A Treatise on Plague dealing with the Historical, Epidemiological, Clinical, Therapeutic and Preventive Aspects of the Disease*, Cambridge University Press, 1905.

The Plague Reconsidered: A new look at its origins and effects in 16th and 17th century England, A Local Population Studies Supplement, 1977.

WU, LIEN-TEH, *A Treatise on Pneumonic Plague*, The League of Nations, Geneva, 1926.

WU, LIEN-TEH., CHUN, J. W. H., POLLITZER, R. and WU, C. Y., eds, *Plague, A Manual for Medical and Public Health Workers*, National Quarantine Service, Shanghai Station, China, 1936.

ZIEGLER, PHILIP, *The Black Death*, Pelican Books.

Secondary works not mentioned in text.

BURNET, MACFARLANE & WHITE, DAVID, *Natural History of Infectious Diseases*, Cambridge University Press, 1972.

CHRONICON ADAE DE USK, A.D. 1377–1421, E. M. THOMSON, ed., Oxford, 1904.

CLEMOW, F. G., *Geography of Epidemic Disease*, Cambridge University Press, 1900.

FOWLER, P. J., ed., *Recent Work in Rural Archaeology*, Moonraker Press, Bradford-on-Avon, 1975.

GALE, A. H., *Epidemic Diseases*, Penguin, London, 1959.

GREENWOOD, Major, *Epidemiology, Historical and Experimental*, Oxford University Press, London, 1932.

GREENWOOD, Major, *Epidemics and Crowd Disease*, Macmillan, New York, 1935.

HALLAM, H. E., *Settlement and Society*, Cambridge University Press, 1965.

HOENIGER, R., *Der Schwarze Tod in Deutschland*, Berlin, 1882.

JOHN, F. M., *The Black Death*, London, 1920.

LECHNER, K., *Das Grosse Sterben in Deutschland*, Innsbruck, 1884.

MULLETT, C. F., *The Bubonic Plague and England*, University of Kentucky Press, Lexington Ky., 1956.

NOHL, J. *Der Schwarze Tod*, Potsdam, 1924.

BIBLIOGRAPHY

PHILIPPE, A., *Histoire de la Peste Noire*, Paris, 1853.

TITOW, J. Z., *English Rural Society*, George Allen and Unwin, London, 1969.

TITOW, J. Z., *Winchester Yields. A study in medieval agricultural productivity*, Cambridge Studies in Economic History, Cambridge University Press, 1972.

RAZI (Al-ḥāwi fi'ṭ-ṭibb), *An Encyclopaedia of Medicine*, Osmania Oriental Publ. Bureau, 1955.

RAZI (Al-ḥāwi fi'ṭ-ṭibb). (1555). *Libellus de peste, de Graeco in Latinum sermonem uersus per N. Macchellum.*

SIGERIST, H. E., *Civilization and Disease*, 3rd edn., University of Chicago Press, 1970.

SLACK, P. A., *Some aspects of epidemics in England 1485–1640*, D. Phil. thesis, Oxford University, 1972.

ZINSSER, H., *Rats, Lice and History*, London, 1943.

Index